THE FAMILY GUIDE TO MEDICAL SCHOOL ADMISSIONS

JANET SNOYER WITH ELYSE PERRUCHON

Disclaimer: The information contained within this Book is strictly for educational purposes. If you wish to apply ideas contained in this Book, you are taking full responsibility for your actions. The authors have made every effort to ensure the accuracy of the information within this book was correct at time of publication. The authors do not assume and hereby disclaim any liability to any party for any loss, damage, or disruption caused by errors or omissions, whether such errors or omissions result from accident, negligence, or any other cause.

First Edition 2021.

Paperback ISBN: 978-0-578-30409-0
Digital ISBN: 978-0-578-30749-7

To Manisha
who taught me all about parenting, and love.

Contents

Acknowledgments

If I knew going into this project how much heart, mind and soul I would need to pour into writing and publishing a book, I would not have felt so impatient with myself over the past eight years since I first felt called to offer this to you. I would still have done it, though, because like so much in our culture, medical school admissions advising is not equitably provided, not equally accessible to all. First, I want to thank everyone who convinced me that advising access is inequitable, so I would become committed to leveling the playing field my way, by sharing all you need to be an advisor to a premed who you love.

I want to thank Cornell University, where I learned most of what I know about premed advising. Three faculty members have given me so much wisdom and generosity of spirit: Bill Crepet, Jeffrey Doyle, and throughout all trials, the ever-supportive Jerry Feigenson.

Thank you to the parents who trusted me with their precious offspring who dared to dream of becoming physicians. I am particularly indebted to the three families who sent me three premeds each (you know who you are). I wish they had more children!

Thank you to every applicant who put their faith in our work together and flew away to medical school to heal the world.

I want to thank all the admissions dean physicians, Robert Witzburg, George Heinrich, Charles Bardes, Valerie Parkas, Steve Gay, Gabe Garcia, Kirsten Lobdell, Clara Callahan, Carol Terregino and others who opened their minds to me so I could learn from them.

Thanks to the hard working admissions directors and deans who sat with me for lunch or coffee, who picked up the phone and answered my questions when they were burning inside me:

Darrell Nabers, Noreen Kerrigan, Gaye Sheffler, Sylvia Robertson, Mercedes Rivero, Carol Teener, Leila Amiri, Juliet Hill, Jen Kimball, Lori Nicolaysen, Liliana Montana, Monica Lopez. There are so many more. You have all taught me so much.

I also want to thank NAAHP and the many advisors who have joined me at meetings and shared their wisdom. Some retired, some gone from this life, all deeply appreciated and their words are woven into mine: David Thurlow, Cha Sook You, Dan Scheirer, Grace Hershman, Caleb Marsh, Robert Rarig, Carol Baffi-Dugan, Glenn Cummings, Nancy Blass, Connie O'Hara, David Verrier, Ellen Snydman, Mariella Mecozzi, Cheire Pereira, Joy Swanson, Jason D'Antonio, Thea Volpe, Robert Schwartz, Julie Chanatry, Kristin McJunkins, Kathleen Kolberg, Jane Cary, Jan Reichard-Brown, Joon Kim, Elba Muñoz, Justin Crowley, Melinda Cohen, Lolita Wood-Hill, Judy Jensvold and Niki Cunningham, just to name a few of those colleagues I most appreciate and respect for so many different reasons.

My family has been a source of strength, delight, diversion and tough love: My sister, Tracey Snoyer and brother, Jeff Snoyer, and his wise spouse, Lynn have found ways to make me know I have a story to tell that the world needs to hear. Friends Paula Winner, Lynn Snoyer (ever-wise paragon of momhood), my sister Dee Key, Rebecca Dolch, Micaela Karlsen, Leslie Ihde, (along with their pets), and Dan Evett, have either fed me regularly, read my work, or both. Dr. Louis Kuchnir has been a kindred spirit from the start.

To the ones most responsible for strengthening and supporting me professionally, I want to give special recognition to: Andrew Simmons, Jennifer Welch, Robert Humbracht.

This book would not have life without the hard work and material contributions of two phenomenal women:

Elyse Perruchon, my co-author, consummate wordsmith, garden designer, reflexologist, wise woman and treasured friend, who has been a constant support and sustainer of my vision, the

Mentoring Alliance and beloved by our applicants.

Finally, I thank my precious, beautiful, smart entrepreneurial daughter, Manisha Snoyer, who got me going, keeps me going and really knows how to hang in there, who has believed in me every step of the way, set me up at the start line, and got us to the finish line with her superb organizational skills, her romantic attachment to the prose and her genuine interest in what her mother does for a living.

Preface

It was a dark and stormy night—and it was cold. I remember that clearly because my cell phone often doesn't receive well inside my house and I went out on the deck to take an unscheduled late night call from MaryBeth Creighton. As the wind howled and my dog peered at me through the sliding glass door from the comfort of the living room, MaryBeth worried out loud.

A month before we met, MaryBeth, a single self-supporting mom, had taken out a second mortgage to send her middle son, Conan, to a post-baccalaureate program to enhance his academic record. She had just learned from her son that the program's institutional letter would not be submitted early enough to give him any leverage in the next admission cycle. MaryBeth worried that Conan's medical school applications would be passed over yet again.

Ella, MaryBeth's youngest, who was a pediatric clinical research coordinator in Manhattan by day and full time member of a modern dance troupe in Queens by night, had retaken the MCAT after studying for six months during her daily subway rides between her two full time activities. MaryBeth had asked Ella again about her MCAT scores which were released two months ago. But Ella told her she "wasn't ready" to see her MCAT score–
–she was having too good a time in NYC and thought it might dampen her spirits. MaryBeth had sold the trees that once filled

the now bleak area behind her house to a timber company to pay for Ella's application fees in the approaching admissions cycle. As my fingers gradually stiffened and lost feeling in the frigid Ithaca winter night, I hopped around the deck offering comfort and counsel to MaryBeth.

What was MaryBeth seeking from me that night? My gut (which provided the body heat for my conversation) sent up a clear message: *Parents need to know what's going on with medical school admissions. They need confidence, reassurance, and validation. Write a guide for parents. Share everything they need to know to be the best advisor possible for their kids.*

And so the idea of this guide was born—to prepare you and your child for the challenges of the medical school admissions process. Just as I know your child will be uniquely qualified to attend medical school after you work through this book together, I feel uniquely qualified to be your guide. Taking turns as a learning strategies counselor, university admissions officer, college success teacher and counselor, institutional health careers committee letter writer, and main advisor at an Ivy League university that sends over 400 applicants to medical school each year, I've advised students on every aspect of the medical and dental admissions cycle. It has all led me to the place I am now, where I can reach over and hold your hand through the anxiety and complexity of medical school admissions.

When I work with applicants, my primary goal is to help them build confidence in themselves by identifying their distinguishing characteristics and strengths. In my experience, anyone can achieve their dream of becoming a doctor if they are willing to tell the truth about themselves and to take the time that they need to build their case for medical school. In my experience, parents want their premeds to succeed, but not at the expense of their zest for living. In my experience, good family communication and support make the trek through challenging times, like the medical school admission cycle, much easier. And finally, in my experience, I've seen the need for this book, *The Family Guide to Medical School Admissions*, so I wrote it.

In *The Family Guide to Medical School Admissions*, I express everything I know (that can be written down) about guiding young healers to achieve their dreams of becoming physicians. My goal is to share the intricacies of the medical school admissions process with the parents and mentors of young healers so families can feel empowered in the journey. *The Family Guide to Medical School Admissions* has four parts.

Part I: Supporting the Dream

The first part is a guide to parenting a person who dreams of becoming a doctor. Good premed parenting differs from what the prevailing wisdom dictates for parenting a young adult in at least two important respects. The first and most important is this: For the period of the application cycle, around 20 months, there is no plan B. It's a full throttle, total surrender, leap into an often mystifying and paradoxical culture posing as a system. The second is that your applicant is allowed to need your support, your money and your inspiration. She is no longer a toddler riding your shoulders and clapping her hands at the summer festival; she's a full grown adult standing on those shoulders, teetering mightily at times, and utterly depending on the steady foundation you provide.

The first part of this book is about building confidence and sustaining it against the many stressors that show up, it's about unobtrusively watching for signs of downheartedness and hopelessness, it's about how your unquenchable love can be one of the most significant factors in helping your offspring reach their dreams. We'll discuss your child's ambitions, what it takes to be a doctor, the ideal medical school admissions scenario, and how you can be good company on the journey.

Part II: Planning the Path to Medical School

Part Two of *The Family Guide to Medical School Admissions is* a detailed guide to the nuts and bolts of the medical school admissions process. It provides facts and insight that you won't find on the internet or in most books on this topic because most writers have not seen this process from the vantage point that I had, when I was the main advisor for a large, socioeconomically and ethnically diverse university. As an admissions advisor continually building relationships with medical schools and admissions staff, I am constantly immersed in information and conversations about medical school admissions criteria, pre-interview and post-interview screening, red flags in candidate applications, and qualities different schools are recruiting for.

In Part Two, I'll explain how to plan and navigate the premed path with your child. We'll discuss the challenges that may arise in high school and college, talking through steps, solutions, and decision points, and how important it is to stay focused on the goal. We'll work through your applicant's preparation options and examine the nuances that distinguish schools and applicants from each other. This section offers steps, solutions and decision points. It gives you the optimal oversight to understand how your child is distinctive, original and ready to become a doctor.

Part III: The Application Cycle

In Part Three of *The Family Guide to Medical School Admissions*, we'll give an overview of the admissions cycle, how an applicant conceives of and learns to articulate their narrative, including writing essays for the primary and secondary application, and matching their strengths to the schools' missions to both choose a list of schools and assess their fit. We explain each step that applicants will encounter.

Part IV: Your Child Applied to Med School: Now What?

In Part Four of *The Family Guide to Medical School Admissions*, we discuss the wind down from the long and arduous application process. When the last essay has been submitted and your child is recovering after their final interview, I'll lead you through what to do while waiting for an answer and how to follow-up with medical schools. We consider each possible outcome, from choosing among acceptances to deciding when to reapply.

For all the premeds who make it to that big dream they worked for since they were five years old when they rescued their first earthworm from the road, and even those few who didn't make it past cadaver lab, we can be pretty sure that they will build meaningful lives for themselves. Given the drive, intelligence, generosity of spirit, diverse array of talents, and just plain abundance of love that set premeds apart, we can count on them to land safely from their leap of faith into the unknown world of medical school admissions. I know your child is these things because I have worked with over 5,000 applicants and found the strengths and the potential in each one. You are not the safety net anymore, but you are definitely holding up your end of it! The safety net is their own resilience, confidence, and incessant yearning to make the world a better place for everybody else: especially you!

1 The Current Landscape

Wanted: 21st Century Physician

Altruistic, compassionate, courageous, intellectually curious, frugal scholar, gifted in history, philosophy, politics, economics, sociology, and psychology. Must have working knowledge of biology, chemistry, physics, and medicine. Physical endurance, emotional maturity, and technical-manual skills sufficient to take apart and reassemble the human body and mind at levels ranging from the micromolecular to the gross are required; must have flexibility to master all knowledge, sift and discard that no longer applicable, while discovering new data at the bench, in clinical practice, in both general and subspecialty medicine. Teaching, counseling, administrative, computer, and budgetary expertise is essential, as is commitment to the disenfranchised. A working knowledge of the law; literary, artistic, and musical talent; and multilingualism is highly desirable. Should be able to prevent and cure disease, including the depredations of advancing age; physical disarray; and spiritual, mental, emotional, and economic illnesses. Will need to function effectively and efficiently in both intensive care units and urban slums. Salary ideally should be no issue, though heavy initial investment by the candidate is required. Benefits variable, depending on the individual's principal source of gratification. This is a 24 hour per day commitment. Should make house calls.

~ Faith T. Fitzgerald, MD

The True Goal

The road to medical school as a series of steps is covered in great detail later in this book. Here we talk about the psychological road. A distinguishing factor of this road is that there is a concrete goal at the end. You and your applicant need to address the question of what this goal actually is. Because you are of the generation that gave birth to the premed you are supporting, as their parent, relative or mentor, you need accurate, nuanced and specific information to help guide your applicant through this long and challenging process.

Who wants to go to medical school? Forgive me: I deliberately asked the wrong question, to distinguish for you, the reader, the true goal from the intermediate one. The correct answer to: Who wants to go to medical school? is "precious few." The right question is: "Who wants to become a doctor?" The goal before your premed is not actually to get into medical school. The goal is to become a physician. To get those MD, DO (or ND) initials, your premed needs the training; no question about it. But if you think that gaining a seat in medical school is the goal, it's really important to reframe that goal now.

One of my heroines is Rachel Naomi Remen, author of **Kitchen Table Wisdom** and **My Grandfather's Blessings**. These books, which were New York Times best sellers for over a decade, tell stories that dotted the life of a physician, told from her perspective as a person who has suffered from a debilitating chronic disease for over 60 years and who rose to become one of the first female pediatricians to train at what is now Weill Cornell Medical School and to serve as Department Head of Pediatrics at Stanford University.

In her later career, Rachel worked exclusively on burnout, or what she calls "compassion fatigue" in physicians. She studied, lectured and provided workshops on this issue, explaining its sources, etiology, course of action and how to reverse it. I have attended several of her workshops, wanting to learn from the doctor attendees as they candidly discuss how their heart for medicine slipped away and to witness them processing adverse, traumatizing events in their career as they learn the work they need to do to reclaim their connection to that deep calling to heal others. I hope that this knowledge will help me in my advising practice to inoculate my premed applicants against this terrible and unexpected condition: to wake up one day and not care about one's patients or one's career at all.

Dr. Remen's books are more often gifted to people than bought for the purchaser's own use. So many people, inspired by her, and by the ubiquitous need they observe, want to help physicians hold on to their hearts and souls, the humanity in medicine. This is your primary and fundamental job as a support person for your premed. You can give them a copy of this book after you have read it yourself, so you may better appreciate what they are up against.

After one of Dr. Remen's workshops, she was saying goodbye to participants who had shared so much of their struggles during the weekend. I waited in line, knowing that I do not strictly belong to their tribe, that I was simply privileged to observe, but I wanted my moment with her. To my delight, Rachel pulled me into a hug. She whispered something in my ear that I will never forget: "Tell your applicants that they are already doctors."

This proved to be one of the most fundamentally wise and useful lessons I have received in my time as a premed admissions counselor/coach/advisor. To you, reader, a person who loves and supports at least one premed, I recommend that you begin now to think of your premed this way, as one who is already a doctor, who just needs the training. The goal for your premed is to become a physician who loves her work, her patients, her colleagues and her life throughout her career as a physician. Getting into medical school is an intermediate goal that you will all want to put in the rearview mirror as soon as possible after it happens!

Perspective and It's All About Plan A

To weather the approximately two years of active candidacy for medical school, the applicant needs perspective on the process and perspective on his chances. This perspective is formed from his assessment of his metrics (MCAT, GPA). Many premeds tell themselves that the metrics are the biggest determinant of their chances, but that's not true. As a parent, you need to be a benign skeptic of that, and ask them not to believe it when they think that. This chart developed by the Dean of Admissions at Boston University School of Medicine and a former officer of the American Association of Medical Colleges, Robert Witzburg, MD with Henry Sondheimer, MD, retired AAMC Senior Director of Student Affairs, will support you in claiming that metrics aren't everything:

Mapping Desirable Physician Traits to Applicant Data.

Physician Trait	Applicant Data Elements
Intellectual ability	Academic record
Commitment to service	History of engagement
Cultural sensitivity	Past behavior
Empathy	Essay, letters of reference
Capacity for growth	Adversities overcome
Emotional resilience	Distance traveled*
Strength of character	Letters of reference, testimonials
Interpersonal skills	Interview, letters of reference
Curiosity and engagement	Life choices

* "Distance traveled" refers to cumulative life experiences — how far one has come in life, rather than physical distance.

[1]

In addition to metrics, medical schools evaluate what the AAMC calls "Experiences and Attributes." Attributes are, in general, the things about an applicant that she is not really responsible for (sex, gender, ethnicity). Experiences are the choices she has made

1 Robert A. Witzburg, MD, and Henry M. Sondheimer, MD April 25, 2013 N Engl J Med 2013; 368:1565-1567 DOI: 10.1056/NEJMp1300411

about how to spend her time outside of class. All these factors go into admissions decisions.

Sometimes parents think that to have "perspective" means that their premed needs to remember there are other health careers besides allopathic medicine (the MD) or osteopathic medicine (the DO), careers in nursing, pharmacy, research, all with doctoral end degrees that give them enormous career latitude. While that's true, most premeds find reminders of that to be deflating. When I met Warren, he was finishing up an admissions cycle where he had six interviews and was rejected from five of those schools after he spent a day meeting with them. His medical school dreams rested on one waitlist, which turned into a rejection at the end of the cycle.

Warren's grandfather, a beloved doctor, had inspired him throughout his life. His parents were pretty disinterested in him and very involved in their own work. They thought he had poor judgment to go into any field that cost so much for the training and took so long before it paid off financially. They had almost completely cut off any emotional contact with him early in his college years. While Warren had little contact with them, he had long weekly conversations with his grandfather. More than anyone, Warren wanted to join his grandfather's profession. He worked at it, earning a 3.98 at a rigorous Ivy League university and scoring in the 97th percentile nationally on the MCAT. A chemistry major, Warren had done research for four years and served as a teaching assistant for organic chemistry in the summers. He was the nicest, smartest, most dedicated guy ever.

Warren's lack of perspective came with the interview. He considered it an afterthought. He expected to put on a suit, show up at the school, answer their questions and get accepted. The schools, it turned out, felt something was off about him. When Warren hired me for his reapplication cycle, I learned this. An introvert, and obviously uncomfortable when attention focused on his achievements, Warren came off as shy. Shyness is easily misinterpreted on interview day as a sign of an interpersonal problem, a social anxiety or phobia. Once a concern like this comes up, it's hard for the admissions committee to see past it. His introverted nature probably factored into his decision to rationalize that it wasn't important to prepare for interviews.

When Warren was rejected from his final school, he found his way to me, and asked me to help him reapply. On the second round, he had 12 interviews and is now a physician in a highly selective residency program. A crisis midway nearly precipitated a second unsuccessful cycle. After his first two interviews, Warren was again waitlisted at both schools. We were working hard on his interview skills at that time. He called his grandfather for comfort. His grandfather replied with what I think of as the standard, Plan B, consolation response. He emphatically assured him he would be just as proud of him if Warren became a pharmacist. Maybe Warren should apply for a pharmacy degree soon.

The next time we met for interview preparation, Warren was monosyllabic in his replies. I began to push for responsiveness and authenticity. He broke down in the tears that had been held back through his whole miserable year and a half of not getting in. He told me how his grandfather counseled him. "Now even he no longer believes in me!" he sobbed.

This—and other similar comments from family members with the best of intentions—is why I counsel parents to leave their Plan B ideas off the stove during the admissions cycle. Do not even put Plan B on the back burner. Deep freeze it. Perspective in the premed ethos means that you are certain he will get in somewhere where he can make his way to becoming as great a doctor as he aspires to be. Recognize that part of the reason you suggest, or want to suggest, Plan B is to soothe yourself during this challenging period.

Warren did not need to know he could enter a different profession. Nor did he need a personality transplant. He did not need a therapist. He needed to learn how to reflect on his life, choices, experiences and aspirations in real time in a real conversation with a medical school faculty member. He needed to learn how to hold up his end of a conversation about himself. His parents did not talk with him. His grandfather was a kind teacher, not a conversant. Warren did not learn the skills he needed at university in lecture courses and the chemistry lab, where he deferred to others.

He did learn these things in time, not overnight. He learned to be himself in the world and the suite of skills he developed to get through the interview and get into medical school will stand him in good stead for a lifetime. After he matriculated, he sent me a card that I treasure and put on my office wall. It says: "Sometimes your only mode of available transportation is a leap of faith. – Margaret Shepard." He also checked in for a few interview prep sessions when he was applying for residency.

Daniel J. Siegel, MD and Tina Payne Bryson, PhD, have published a great book called **The Power of Showing Up (2020).** They include this sage wisdom about what it means to be a supportive parent, which applies so well to serving the premed journey as a family member. They explain that the term "support" contains what they call "the 'Four S's' – helping them feel 1) safe – where they feel protected and sheltered from harm; 2) seen – where they know you care about them and pay attention to them as they really are; 3) soothed – where they know you'll be there for them when they're hurting; and 4) secure – which develops from the other S's so they trust you to predictably help them feel 'at home' in the world." Solving problems with a Plan B is not listed here because your job is to support and serve, not to fix problems over which you have no control.

Validation and Encouraging Resilience

Your premed also needs to cultivate a willingness to move on when unexpected things happen, when bad things happen, and when nothing happens. This may take encouragement from you. You sense her need to validate the immediate moment of distress, but you keep your own perspective, which is always that this event does not portend the end of the world, nor will it keep them out of medical school. It's good to keep in mind something the Dalai Lama, the spiritual leader of Tibet, tells his own followers: *Remember that not getting what you want is sometimes a wonderful stroke of luck.*

While having a big bad thing happen can feel like a pothole on the road to medical school, in some respects, the worst part of applying to medical school is when nothing happens, which is most of the time. While he is kept busy during May to July of his application year, composing supplemental essays that easily amount to over 50 pages of writing, he receives only auto-generated messages, if he's lucky, from a handful of the schools where he applied. It's normal for nothing to happen, and it's normal for him to feel that he has waited long enough. The trouble is that it usually takes longer to hear back than feels right or fair–or even like the admissions offices run a competent process to the interested onlooker.

He applies in June, application is complete in July, and he is offered an interview in January. Typical. Seven long months without a bite. The more you expect this, the better you will be able to handle it. It's hard to talk about how nothing is happening, but you should bring this up every month or so with your premed so he knows that he is not alone in the agony of not hearing, not knowing and not receiving any response at all from the medical school. Simply let him know that you are in this waiting game with him and that it sucks! (Even though you can console yourself by thinking: "that's life.")

The stress that medical school admissions engenders is real. You will feel it and your applicant will feel it. And you can both handle it. It's important to see it for what it is. At any point in the process, stress can turn into contained panic. It happened to Shannon when she bolted out of her second MCAT administration, mid test, because she just couldn't think. It happened to Sam after he submitted his AMCAS primary application and began to loathe his personal statement. (He was accepted to Harvard and Stanford with that statement, so how pathetic could it have been?) It happened to Travis when he found the faculty physician scientist interviewer he had just spent an hour talking with, was zipping down his fly at the adjacent urinal in the men's room. Travis later joyously accepted a seat at that medical school. It happens when the MCAT scores come back, when the first rejection email arrives, when college-aged romantic partners are disloyal or unfaithful or just act like jerks.

Medical student wellbeing is a topic you can learn a lot about on the internet, including how the culture of medical education affects it, and how you can assuage its potentially destructive effects on our premeds. This takes only the one resource that abundantly flows without stopping between you and them: love. The application cycle will give you a preview of the systemic cultural mores that your applicant will need to learn to face and manage without losing—or worse—sacrificing that precious inner healing spirit. You will learn how to guide your budding physician to follow the core mandate of physician mentors since the time of Aeschylus in Prometheus Bound: "Physician: Heal thyself." And you will be able to give them a core tenet of your own: "Be yourself."[2]

Arguing With Reality

Byron Katie is a contemporary thought leader who has realized some major epiphanies about modern life. I heartily recommend you to her books. She has a pithy brilliance about her and one of my favorites is her definition of stress: "Stress is caused when a person engages in a futile argument with reality."

My applicant, Jeremy, wanted to stay at his undergraduate university and attend its medical school. It was something he really pined after. Months after submitting his application, and getting interviews at other medical schools, he became increasingly frantic. I agreed to call the Director of Admissions

---

2 "Like an unskilled doctor, fallen ill, you lose heart and cannot discover by which remedies to cure your own disease." Also, variants of this are found in the Books of Genesis and Luke in the Bible. Accessed 12/16/19 here: https://www.theoi.com/Text/AeschylusPrometheus.html

to see if any movement was forthcoming on his application, an action that I truly loathe. I really like this admissions officer, but I don't like feigning any pretense of putting my thumb on the scale. We talked. She told me he was a great applicant, which I already knew. She looked his materials over and cited his many assets. "He's great, Janet. It's just that he's a little tiny bit less great than the people we are inviting to interview this year."

I knew that she was speaking in her way for a committee that had already decided to reject Jeremy without an interview. Now it became my problem to continue to advise Jeremy well. Would I dutifully repeat those words to him? I couldn't. They would injure his confidence. How could I guide him through this reality but tell the truth? I decided to tell him that the committee had reviewed him once and weren't going to notify him for some time. That way they would have a chance to revisit his application should their class size permit it. I told him not to hold out great hope, based on the impression I got from the conversation.

Somehow Jeremy managed to deal with this news in a way that made him more resolute in the interviews he had. He was able to stop the obsessive thinking in his head: *Maybe today I will hear from them, maybe if I send them more information, maybe if I find a new letter to add to my file. Maybe if I make myself more appealing, they will interview me. Maybe not,* he told himself, *in fact, probably not.* And when his best friend at school was invited to interview at their medical school, and offered a seat, Jeremy just shrugged and moved on.

As an advisor, I prefer to stay in the background and let the medical schools make their decisions without interrogation from me. I try to be a fly on the wall and study them, like a detective, trying to figure out what they want, and what turns them off to applicants. As a parent, your perspective is limited. You may have only one cycle with one applicant (that's plenty!) and you have to stay in the background. Admissions people at medical schools scorn any parent who wants to interact with them and stereotype those parents harshly, as people who have raised an overly dependent child. Since you cannot become directly involved, it's best that you let go of any such fantasies.

How can a parent observe the stress and discern if it is making the applicant stronger, if she can handle it, if it is overwhelming her or damaging her chances? And how can you protect yourself from absorbing the stress you observe in your premed? One way to deal with both of these concerns is to ask yourself some trenchant questions. What is the conclusion that you or your premed reaches as a result of the stressors? Does she say: *Now I will never get into medical school?* Do you say: *Is this med school thing really worth the time and money we are pouring into it?* If you start to believe these thoughts, you are amping up the stress: waging an argument with reality.

It amazes me sometimes to realize the power of one thought. Byron Katie's advice is not to believe most of what you think. The one question to ask your premed or yourself when you have thoughts that sound like you are certain that a stressful situation portends a dream-crushing failure to become a doctor is: *Do I actually believe that thought?*

If the answer is no, it ought to be pretty easy to chuck it and let the stress tamp down on its own. If the answer is yes, ask again: *Do I actually and honestly, really believe that thought is true?* Sooner or later you will get to no. The reason you get to no is simple. Thoughts that arise out of crises and stress are not facts. They are not observations. They are the opposite. They are false beliefs. The sky is not falling, Henny Penny.

This is the simplest and most fundamental way to maintain your perspective. This is how you heal yourself to be the best support system ever. Question all thoughts. Question false beliefs. Now you are ready to support your premed in becoming the physician they dream to one day be.

2 Communication: How to Be Good Company on the Journey

Is medical school the best career choice for your offspring? Medical school preparation takes considerable time—and you don't need me to tell you that it's not the ideal career for everyone. Because your premed ought to know the less-than-ideal aspects, clinical observation and engagement are non-negotiable elements of a complete application. If you asked most premeds how they know this is the best, or the ideal choice for them, they cannot easily answer. In fact, they resist the question. When I prepare applicants for their first interview, an essential question is: *Why do you want to become a doctor?* Their first response is nearly always: *I hate that question.* They don't know where to start, where to go, and certainly a true response has no natural endpoint. They become engulfed in the chasm between the obvious and the wordless depths, between what they think the admissions committee wants them to present and their most authentic, real-time response.

A life in medicine is something they feel called to. It emanates from the depths of their being, a place they rarely if ever look into voluntarily. What they can and do articulate well is what we might call the unacceptability of "Plan B," as I discussed in an earlier chapter: No matter what obstacles, challenges and even insults and rejections pop up on the path, most premeds cannot and will not envision doing anything else with their lives.

Often family members mutely accept this puzzling and unsatisfying explanation, not wanting to add to the undertow that applicants already feel. They know their applicant and they have seen the steadfast dedication throughout their lives. Nevertheless, you can ask good questions, when the timing is just right, to elicit responses that will help them to better articulate and to justify why medical school is the best career choice for them. This is the positive spirit and productive energy with which you undertake guiding your premed to respond to the question lurking behind *Why do you want to become a doctor?* That question is: *Why is medical school the best career choice for you?*

I suggest you use the productive exercise below to pose this question.

> *Let's work on how to respond to the question of why you want to become a doctor. I am going to ask you a question that gets at why you have devoted your one young life to your mission of becoming a doctor. I will ask you the exact same question fifteen times. The question is: "Why is a medical career the best choice for you?" Each time you answer, I will wait a few seconds, then say: "Thank you." Then we will look with kindness at each other, take a deep breath, and I will ask again.*

Document the responses you hear, either by writing, engaging a scribe who is just there to listen and support, or by recording the conversation. Recording and transcribing are so useful. It gives your applicant a chance to hear themselves, and continue to generate better responses. After this exercise, you can just sit with them. I don't think giving feedback or advice is the best way to debrief. Instead, just ask them how that was and what responses felt most true for them. Just be attentive, grateful, open, honest and quiet; don't try to be wise and helpful, certainly not correcting, rewording or suggesting. They need to know that you trust them to get to the best response themselves and that you think they are enough just as they are with the responses that the question elicited.

You can use recording, both audio and video, as a tool in guiding your aspirant. Many people do not like watching or listening to themselves initially, but it's a good practice. In time, one becomes habituated. When you and your progeny watch the video together, your roles as judge and their roles as self-critics will soften. The recording is a record; it's evidence and a good place to start.

Because I work remotely with nearly all my advisees, long before the coronavirus beset us all, I developed a system of videorecording applicants responding to an individualized set of questions that enhance their reflective capacities, bolster their confidence and point out places where we need to strengthen their resolve and expression of their goals. This has been so helpful to establish a record they can view as often as they wish, with whomever they want, to polish, refine and authenticate their responses, both verbally and non-verbally, through seeing their own body language.

As I mentioned, some applicants feel squeamish in the beginning about watching themselves, but the strategy grows on them. They even like to watch their videos alone in their hotel rooms as they get dressed for interview day. It soothes them to see themselves responding in an environment where they feel safe and supported, and allows them to imagine interview day that way. If you make this recording a common practice early on and use it regularly, they will come to see it as an invaluable tool in polishing their performance for the all-important medical school interview.

Whose Dream Is This Anyway?

Most families, if they really examine their motives in the privacy of their own minds, will find that they have some mixed feelings about this dream. Of course you are proud of them. Of course you love telling your friends that your offspring is planning on medical school. When so many young adults are losing their way, yours has a path, a plan, a safe, sustainable and altruistic future. It is really a huge family achievement.

While you can support it in the big picture, you also may literally feel despair watching your offspring navigate the more punishing aspects of this path and want instinctively to protect them from all that. Sometimes it's convenient to question the other adults who play a role in guiding your offspring along this path. Is the college doing its job? Is the prehealth advisor any good? Is the boss mean? You naturally want to talk with these people, but they all shut you out. When you do reach out, you may feel that they are utterly dismissive of your concerns and consider you to be the problem. You are the snowplow, the helicopter, the out-of-line, ignorant, irrational pain in the neck. It shouldn't be this way, but usually it is.

Parents do not get the respect and consideration they need and deserve. I wrote this book because I think differently about the vital, collaborative role you have in supporting your own medical school aspirant's dream (despite any very understandable, private, mixed feelings you may harbor about this dream or the shocking demand on your financial resources). This book will show you the mindset you need to be valuable and essential company with all the other mentors and gatekeepers who have a say in the matter of whether your offspring gets into medical school. It will also provide expertise and information you are unlikely to find anywhere else. Information like this belongs in a book that you hold in your hands and filter through your own sensibility.

In addition to supporting the big picture, while you support and celebrate the small steps and milestones, you may worry about the larger picture ahead: the future of healthcare and its treatment of doctors. Maybe you, at some point, will compare your own work history to the one you anticipate for your offspring. You may not feel comfortable about yourself deep down, when you know your offspring's status in the world will so eclipse your own. If you have been successful and achieved recognition for your career, you may worry that your offspring is attempting this medical career path in order to live up to your standards rather than forging their own path. Or you may think it's fine for them to be motivated by your expectations while wondering deep down if they will ever feel they have accomplished that, because you yourself grew up under the same conditional love and never felt you were able to satisfy your parents, until the day came where you just didn't care anymore.

Then there's the physical wellbeing of your offspring. Will her ovaries still be able to produce your grandchildren when there's a moment for mating and breeding to be found in this slog to doctorhood?[3] Will his depression stay managed during sleepless nights on call and anxious studying for the countless exams? Will they leave us behind, as they have no control over where they live during residency and no time to stay in touch in a meaningful way? Will our friends and their friends from the neighborhood retreat from them, assuming that they think they are now "better than us?"

It's really healthy to talk this over with your applicant. It's not so easy to find the time, space, will, and knowhow to conduct this conversation. Here are some questions to sprinkle into the conversation, to help you clarify some of the emotional undertow you both feel.

- In what respects would you say you are now an independent adult, taking care of your needs in the different areas of your life? How have we facilitated or hindered that?
- Are we supporting you in the most valuable way possible through this application process?
- Is there any area that you would like us to stay out of, or become more involved in?

---

3 On a side note, one of my former applicants now in medical school told me that she knew nine medical student women whose parents paid for them to have their eggs frozen before they started medical school.

- Do our hopes for you ever get in the way of you realizing your own hopes, whether they are similar or different?
- Who do you trust the most in your application planning and execution?
- Do you want to write your applications without my input?
- What contributions would you like me to make to your application cycle?
- Is there any area of your application you are worried or anxious about that you would like to share with me? Do you want me just to listen or to give you my own thoughts?

What's My Role Anyway?

In looking over the questions I suggested above, you will note that some of them ask you to give your applicant the chance to define your role in this process. When Gina got a C+ on her first organic chemistry exam, she was devastated. She told me her mom knew just what to do. She said: *That sucks! Tell me all about it.* And when Gina had run out of rant, her mom said: *Thank you for letting me know. I love you, honey.* And they said goodbye. That was the ideal role at that moment.

Don't jump into the thinking that you need to read everything you can find on the internet to make you the instant expert advisor. Whatever role you assume, your applicant is likely to interpret in a way that may be very different from your actual motives. If you over-edit their essays, they may think you impugn that they are not effective writers. If you tell them a gap year is a bad idea for their long-term future, they may think you want to rush them so you can free yourself of parental responsibility sooner (as if you could). They may think you won't support them in their application cycle if they delay. They may think you actually believe that their learning machinery will become rusty and obsolete if it is put to other uses for a year between college and medical school.

Your role is to do some personal reflection about your own motives, and then hold them up to the light of day to see which of your motives deserves expression in the application process. When you are not sure, ask the applicant to guide you. They may feel a little awkward with that role reversal, but in the end, it will accomplish what you most want. They will trust you and know that you are there to bear witness to this process, available, accessible, resourceful and responsive. That's your role.

Being a Positive Influence

How do you stay positive when things aren't going well or going at all? We all have different ways of communicating optimism, pessimism, and for that matter, apathy and disinterest. Due to the intrusion of screen culture, our tolerance for distracted communication is at an all time high. You and your premed need to give each other undistracted time when the subject is the medical school application cycle. That discipline alone, modeling it for your family, will make you a positive influence.

The single most frequent reason a parent calls me is impatience with the process. *Should I be worried?* Between November and March, that's why applicants contact me too. *What should I do?* They—parents and their premeds—try not to talk to each other about the lingering uncertainty caused by hearing nothing. Since humans all too frequently interpret no news as bad news before they try to reason themselves into a neutral or positive outlook, I am glad they reach out to me, if only to voice their private thoughts and watch them shrivel in the light of day.

When uncertainty about a monumental decision is accompanied by fear of loss, confidence erodes. The word confidence has the roots "con" which means coming together and "fid," which means faith. Confidence is the state of coming together in faith. Uncertainty frays and undermines confidence. It's really not productive nor is it helpful to share your uncertainty directly with your premed during the cycle. Afterwards, when you debrief, no problem. To be a positive influence, you need to catch yourself misinterpreting waiting as a bad omen. It's just not true that being made to wait is a negative sign. If your applicant does express their suffering at the long wait, do not commiserate. There's a big difference between these two simple replies: *I am also worried.*

How can we fix this? versus: *We expected this. We can handle it.* Go for the latter.

Family Issues in Supportively Raising a Premed

If your premed has been raised by more than one parental figure (and so many family configurations abound these days), you are used to having perhaps diverging takes on advising your progeny. The medical school application process presents a few dimensions for disagreement. First: how much you know versus how much your co-parent knows. How much you care, how attached you are to the outcome, how much your premed listens to you versus them. Often the premed sees the diverging wisdom of parents, parental figures, or mentors as falling along a major fault line: subjective or objective, nurturing or authoritative, emotional or rational, supportive or intrusive. Once you characterize each other or are characterized this way, the suggestions you make, advice you give, and reactions you have to setbacks and achievements are viewed through those rigid lenses.

Let's take the situation of when your premed gets an interview and then is waitlisted. The subjective parent sympathizes and validates their disappointment and uncertainty. The objective parent recommends action, like the letter of intent technique they read about on the internet. The subjective parent diminishes the objective parent's advice as poorly timed, ineffective or unethical. The objective parent diminishes the subjective parent's sympathy as encouraging helplessness or dependency to no fruitful end. The person at the receiving end of all this wants support, but also wants reliable information. Of course you should comfort your offspring, but only provide information when you are absolutely sure it's useful. This is hard to know if it's your first time through a 21st century admissions cycle.

A wise family unit locates its authorities early on in the cycle and trusts them to talk things over before weighing in. Even an overly strong nurturing reaction to a temporary setback like a waitlist notification that follows an interview decision can fray confidence. It can make an applicant feel like their worst fears are actually valid. And likewise, the rational response to do something, send something, read the message boards online about the experience of other applicants, can prompt you to give very unwise counsel at a critical time to your applicant. It's fun, perhaps, for you, to be the one voicing the information, but in doing so, you can risk their alienation and withdrawal from you. This could prohibit you from being the source of unconditional support that they truly need in their lives.

Time, Stress and Energy Management

The medical school admissions cycle is not something to bounce along, taking things as they come. The applicant needs a clear path and well-prepared ground. You wouldn't predict that you could stick an avocado pit in a highway dirt triangle in the harsh climate of New York City and expect it to bloom and bear fruit once, much less perennially. The medical school admissions cycle can bear the analogy to a garden. What you sow is what you will reap. You need to start with hardy plantings selected for resilience. Just as gardens thrive in optimal environments below and above the ground, and flourish with proper nutrients, water, and sunshine, applicants need sleep, exercise, nutritious food, and well-developed management skills to optimize stress and energy. They also need to know that you and their family are okay.

Corinna grew up the youngest in a family of four children that had the tradition of weekly family dinners at the homes of her maternal and paternal grandparents, respectively. During a particularly rugged academic term, piled high with club leadership, organic chemistry, biochemistry and a 15-hour weekly commitment to her research lab, when she was also studying for a scheduled late spring MCAT administration, her maternal grandmother, with whom she loved to bake and knit throughout childhood, fell ill and was institutionalized, barely clinging to life. Her paternal grandfather, a physician she had always revered, was diagnosed with pancreatic cancer and underwent chemo and radiation. Corinna's parents and older brothers, two in medical school, agreed that they needed to protect Corinna from the grief and worry they felt. They decided she should not know of these events, even when her beloved grandmother died and they held her funeral, without Corinna.

When Corinna decided to surprise her family by taking the bus home and showing up at the weekly family dinner hosted by her paternal grandmother, she was shocked to find her grandpa weak and gaunt. She texted her mom at the dinner table and learned the rest of the family news, that her mom's mother had been sick and died. Corinna's stable, resourceful management of her life, her stress, and her outlook was shattered. She felt betrayed, outraged, misunderstood and submerged in oceanic grief. What her brothers and parents had framed as "protection" was actually a set up for trauma, which is, seen from Corinna's perspective, a level of stress that can't be borne, much less managed.

Rule #1 in dealing with a premed is that you need to tell them when people they love are injured or ill. As Corinna put it, she could have comforted her mother and father instead of having to confront them with the news that they were not protecting her, but setting her up for a loss from which she would not soon recover. So many premeds found their inspiration to practice medicine while they sat by the bedside of an ailing loved one, watching and questioning the doctors and nurses and ably occupying the role of a wise and informed presence for their families. They are not children to be protected; they are on the road to becoming doctors who have a need to know.

It is useful to think of time and energy management during the medical school admissions cycle as a muscle group often subject to overuse injury, rather than conjuring up the image of a color-coded and overfilled desk calendar. The energy management muscle group is conditioned in the undergraduate years, so it can be adapted to the admissions cycle. The task of the admissions cycle is to develop a robust narrative which is then retrofitted to written (primary and secondary applications) and verbal (interview) expressions of the applicant's preparation, readiness, value to the school's mission, and informed commitment to a life in medicine. The narrative is tailored to the criteria that admissions screeners, interviewers and committee members use to steadily shrink the applicant pool: from interview potential to interview invite to waitlisted and accepted.

Applicants often have great difficulty estimating the preparation time they need on the verbal section of the MCAT: Critical and Analytical Reasoning, or CARS. Weak writing and superficial reading skills can show up to doom them in that section, something they may not even realize as they methodically plod through the passages given in practice tests and exercises. CARS is the hardest section for applicants to prepare for, particularly those raised in multilingual families, just as the essays are a huge hurdle for most.

Undergraduate universities find it challenging to allocate resources necessary to teach writing to a mastery level. It takes curious, well-trained and energetic instructors to teach writing, and the lack of investment in writing curriculum, particularly at large universities for non-humanities students is obvious to those who review the essays applicants to medical schools compose. All this is to say that applicants often have little to no idea of how long they will need to draft, refine and polish the essays that they will submit to medical schools as part of their application. This can make energy and time management daunting. It can also result in unimpressive, "good enough" essays that don't really give the admissions office what it needs to move the applicant along to the next selection pool.

To prime your applicant for productive and effective energy and time management through the writing-intensive part of the admissions cycle, you can offer to look at what's ahead of them and help them to create a personalized timeline, a set of wiggly deadlines that point toward the goal of completing secondary applications by July 1 of the calendar year. You can find generic timelines on the internet to start with, but they need to be retrofitted to the other tasks your premed has taken on between November 15 and June 30.

An online, cloud-based spreadsheet works great. I use Google Sheets with my applicants because it's easy to share, and for all interested parties to view, comment, and edit. I recommend putting the calendar dates as columns and the tasks as rows. Tasks should be bundled into groups that occur nearly simultaneously in the cycle: something like the table below, although each of the tasks on the figure can be even further broken down into multiple line items.

Overview of The Medical School Application Timeline

Jan	Feb	Mar	Apr	May	Jun	Jul	Aug	Sep	Oct	Nov	Dec	Jan	Jan	Feb	Mar	Apr	May	Jun	Jul	Aug
Draft Primary Application Essays (Personal Statement)																				
	Request Letters of Recommendation																			
		Request and Review Transcripts																		
				Submit Primary																
					Transcripts Are Verified															
						Submit Secondary Applications														
								Complete Interviews												
										Send Updates to Medical Schools										
															Choose Your Medical School					
																Orientation, Financial Aid, Housing				
																			Start Medical School	

Energy management is based on the principle that it can take you half the time to complete a complex activity at an optimal point of the day than it takes at a suboptimal one. I am writing these words first thing in the morning because if I were to procrastinate until after dinnertime, I would write one third as much in an hour and it would take twice the editing to express it in the way I hope to inform you.

You can help with energy management by applying the observations you have made of your applicant's energy cycle through the day, their biorhythm. Many premeds have almost unnatural stamina, focus and tenacity. Their mothers marvel at the hours they sit at the kitchen table on school breaks poring over their MCAT books. Just remember that the time they sit in the chair may not be as productive as it seems to the observer. This is a human body, not a machine, and naturally, energy and attention will wax and wane.

People who stretch themselves to the limit, whether it be physically, intellectually or any other way, often drop healthy habits along the way. They thus lose a sense of the best working equation for personal balance and true optimal productivity. You don't have to accept these varying notions of "normal." Instead, sit down with a warm cuppa' something and inquire with your premed about what really is their best balance of nutrition, exercise, sleep and learning.

Here are some good questions to guide your aspiring physician to gain mastery of energy management:

- What is their biorhythm for the tasks that currently fill their days?
- When do they write best?
- When are they at their mental learning peak?
- How long can they write before the function declines—or it takes longer to put thoughts down?
- How much sleep do they need and between what hours?
- What happens to their cognitive function when they haven't had enough sleep?
- Have they ever tried quiet meditation to clear their mind before writing or studying?
- What foods give them energy?
- Which foods and at what time make them more sluggish or sleepy?
- Are they hydrating throughout the day?
- How long is their attention span for passive review? For answering practice questions?

Encouraging Reflection

A good practice for you, practically speaking, is to sit down with yourself, or sit down with a life partner who also loves your offspring. Sit with your spouse or your sibling or someone else who has been with you, such as a good friend who raised his children coincident with your raising yours. Sit with each other, each with a piece of paper and a pen. You will take turns scribing so you have a record of the conversation. Ask your exercise partner this question: *What are the most delightful aspects of your child, whose spirit you have come to know over the years?* You write down what the person said about their child and say only: *Thank you*—no commentary. And then they can ask you to answer the same question about your own child, and they will write down your answer. *What are the most delightful aspects of Herman's spirit?*

Alternating, continue to pose each of your respective questions over and over exactly the same way 20 times. Each time you ask, you'll get the opportunity for a new insight. Process the exercise. As you read aloud what your exercise partner said about their own child, chime in at that point with things that you have also seen in their child. If you cannot do it in person, use video software and transcribe as you go or later. I recommend transcribing in real time.

Later, you can sit down with your premed and say: *Have you ever thought about my spirit?* Ask them what they think is the finest quality or the most positive qualities they have observed in what you can call your "spirit"—and you don't really want to define what that word, spirit, means for people. A good working definition for spirit is: the source of their inspiration. You can say to them, "Is there a way in which I, as your parent, have inspired you?" "Is there a way in which your aunt or your mentor have inspired you?"

Make sure that they know you're not looking for compliments. You're asking them to show you that they see things in you. This may not be an ease-ful conversation, but it will be a good way to facilitate what might be even more challenging for them, to talk about their own qualities of spirit. You will be prepared for that. The things they say about you are likely to be qualities they themselves evince and then you can share with them everything your exercise partner and you said for them to chew over—if or when they find themselves at a loss. Try to go beyond what you might usually talk about or share in an explicit way. And once you get them in this game, your conversation will rise to a new level of sharing and intimacy.

I promise you that many applicants write about their parent's spirit in their personal statements. *My father has inspired me in his tenacity as a lawyer to always serve justice. My mother has inspired me as a schoolteacher in the story she brings home about the transformation she's seen in the inner city children she serves.*

Honestly, you may not be very proud of yourself because of the way you see at this point that your own life has turned out. Maybe this is because you still see unhelpful conditioning from your own childhood, habits you may despair of, or even addictive behaviors that you haven't been able to rid yourself of. Maybe you feel that the level of work in the world that you've risen to, your impact on the world, is not a source of pride. Nevertheless, within the unit of your family or in your mentorship of your offspring, you will most definitely find ways in which you inspire your premed. *My mother has struggled with depression for as long as I can remember, but when we really need her, she always finds a way to be there for us.*

Once you get them thinking about that, if your timing is well-chosen, you could pull out your sheet of paper, and say, *well, these are the things about your spirit that inspire me.* This will almost certainly prompt a talk about those qualities. And in some ways, it takes some discipline to make this worthwhile, because it can sound a little bit like bare naked flattery, and just boasting about each other in a way. I can't tell you how often I'll hear parents say something like *I really admire my child because she never quits. She's so dedicated.* And then what comes after that really great morsel of information that I need to know is, *but I'm just her mother. I'm probably biased.* This pervasive sense of what I call the "humblebrag" gets in the way of spiritual expression. Who but you yourself is actually whispering to you that your admiration and love for your children is biased or in some way, not accurate or not true because they're your children? I find that point of view frustrating when I hear it, because I want to hear the great things about your child; you know things nobody else does. I'm sure that I can trust that the qualities you cite are there.

Those aspects of character, temperament and *modus operandi* may not show up in our routine advising conversations, yet my job is to help them elicit and learn to express them verbally and in writing.

This kind of exercise encourages self-reflection. And that's something that a lot of young people don't have time for, are not encouraged to do and often don't really discover till they get into their application process. They embody qualities that they have taken completely for granted. Because while they may be hard workers, for example, they will say: *Well, if you're not a hard worker, you will never get into medical school, so I made myself into a hard worker.* They take no credit for the fact that they were able to will themselves to work so hard.

In the course of a safe and low-key conversation that is built on the foundation of the exercises cited above, your offspring can bring up the many good qualities that she embodies, which should be recorded during the conversation, either by you or another parent or friend as a notetaker, or by using a recording software on your phone or other computing device. You review the notes by naming each one of those qualities in a word or two or three, or maybe a sentence. Just be brief. And you can then ask for good stories, which will drive the narrative they share in their applications: *How has your prodigious capacity for hard work shown up in the things that you've chosen to pursue in your life?*

Your offspring has chosen to pursue college, to be a college student, and do four years of college academic work. Paradoxically, if you claim that this was their choice, they might look at you with astonishment. You have both taken it so much for granted that they would go to college that it doesn't seem like a choice to them, but it certainly was. It was a choice to stick it out through some tough times. Nearly all premeds face those tough times. So another way that you can encourage reflection, and the way that medical schools do it, is to regularly inquire about their challenges.

They are also asked about adversity and about problems arising from dysfunctional team work. Medical schools do not ask about that to dip into, or trigger shame on the part of the applicant. They ask about it because that helps them to understand the spirit of the applicant and how resilient and adaptable they are. It is about how they solve problems and how they overcome things. When you ask the question of how life challenged them this week, you are teaching your child to see challenges as normal, to talk intelligently and dispassionately about the obstacles they experience.

Reflection is a really important quality to encourage in your applicant. It might be helpful for you to even join them. You could allot yourself a short period of self-reflection every day. That period of self-reflection can take many different forms. One form that it can take is to write in a journal, simply to think about what happened during the day. Encourage them not to see their life like a movie that they are passively experiencing. It may feel, on first thought, that they go to class and sit there passively and then go to a student activity and sit there passively and then go to the gym and walk on the treadmill for an hour, passively. Ask them how they got involved in these daily events, how they reached out and activated their inner qualities in order to make that experience all that they hoped it would be.

Often people write in their personal statement about a nursing home encounter with someone who is different from them. Usually it's somebody who is older, sicker and not as well connected to the world as they are, and the person is not very communicative, might even be kind of mean, or might have a reputation for being mean. The applicant is volunteering, shadowing, or visiting the institution where this person is residing. The applicant cites an interaction with that person, which leads to a very rewarding breakthrough for that patient or resident. The two have a lovely conversation where your applicant sees the person light up and the applicant walks away feeling incredibly pleased that they evoked that in another person.

But then when they walk away, do they really know what they did that lit up that other person? That's really worth talking about, not telling them, not leading the witness—but listening with appreciative inquiry: *What do you think enabled you to connect to a person who everyone else thinks is a stodgy old curmudgeonly mean person? What was it that made them feel safe and know that you are on their side? What qualities did you bring—and don't just think about the verbal, the things you said. It's the nonverbal. It's not just the things that you say; it's how you say them and how you are. When you walk in the room, do you sit down? Right away, do you get at eye level with a person who might be confined to a bed or do you stand over them? Do you lean in, do you make eye contact, do you laugh at their jokes?*

When you engage in this way to communicate with your premed, you are building their confidence from the ground up. Parental praise, while easily lavished, does not in itself build confidence. Many other adults, peers and authority figures have crowded the space in your child's life of which you were once, many years ago, the sole occupant. Parental praise cannot dispel the voice of the inner critic that so many life experiences have installed on auto-pilot in the privacy of their mind.

Building Confidence

Confidence is an interesting subject. Because confidence, in my experience, really does wax and wane in the premed. We need it to be strong and persistent for them to sustain a career as a physician. Remember, as I noted earlier, when you think about the word confidence, you find it has a very interesting root structure. The central letters of the word, *fid,* is Latin for faith. So confidence, at its core, is about faith. It's not about what you have in front of you. It's about what comes next, and how you feel about it. The prefix *con* means coming together, and has to do with collecting. The suffix, *ence,* means "the state of." So confidence is achieving the state of coming together in faith, and aligning oneself with a predisposition to come together and have faith. Thus, when a person lacks confidence, it's usually because something real or imagined has happened recently that has made them sort of come apart, to dissolve. What is causing the coming apart is usually something that didn't go right in their premed path that makes them feel that maybe they won't even get to go to medical school.

Diffidence is an antonym for confidence, and it has come to infer a kind of shy presentation of self. Diffidence means to diverge from a state of faith in the unseen. Diffidence is rooted in self-doubt, uncertainty, and self-criticism. We don't want the applicant to think that these feelings, even based as they are in real setbacks, are true. Diffidence is based on a rationalization of a negative past experience. Confidence is based on a healthy and optimistic faith in the future that things will work out in the ways that really matter.

I've seen diffidence creep into a premed's habitual way of seeing the world. It happens when he studies for the MCAT, takes a practice test and does not earn a strong enough score. I've seen this happen when a grade comes back below an A-. The student fears that a C grade, or even B grades will shut the gate to medical school. I've seen this happen after an interview, when the applicant wasn't sure how well he did or feels like he didn't show up like he should have and therefore, he is not going to get into medical school. All these downer times, all these little troughs our premeds get into during this process of going through being vetted in so many ways, send the message that maybe medical school is not going to work out, and this is a very painful prospect to contemplate.

Our premeds need to have a way to come together in confidence, to come together in faith that this is going to work out. Parents play an instrumental role in helping their offspring essentially pull themselves together in faith. I have learned along the way, that some of the knee jerk reactions parents have, which they express with the best of intentions to their applicants, really just make things worse.

So here are some ways, some messages you don't want to give to your child when his spirit is raw and out there, and his faith that this is going to happen feels like it's flying apart. Number one is you don't blame the source of the problem, such as:

The MCAT is ridiculous. It's too hard, it's too long. There are not enough administrations scheduled. They're just trying to weed you out. They don't see how great you are. Why do they put so much faith in a standardized test? Why do they reduce you to a number?

All those words and messages can make you feel like you're being supportive, but what you're doing is criticizing an institution that they just really have no choice but to engage with. They have to take the MCAT, so while your feisty criticism may feel good to you, even to them at the time, it subtly encourages them to complain and blame, which does no good, and serves to erode confidence when they need it the most.

Another robust victim of criticism is the teacher. A college teacher, they may claim, isn't a good teacher or doesn't give good tests or doesn't give good feedback or doesn't take enough time to explain things and that's why your applicant thinks that their grade was low. Don't encourage that. Don't support that. You can listen to it, but don't chime in and criticize the teacher further.

Many years ago, a child who I was close to, a 12 year old girl, developed anorexia. She had to be hospitalized and it was very, very scary for all of us. Her mom and dad were asked to attend some pretty painful and mystifying therapy sessions about the quality of love they offered her. While the child felt really safe in the hospital, she also felt quite vulnerable because she was hospitalized for not eating and everyone was watching her eating and exercising and tracking her self-report of her body image.

The therapist encouraged the child to tell her parents how she thought that they could help her better to recover. When she did, the therapist watched how the parents responded. Naturally, the parents were really, really hurt to discover their psychological contribution to the development of her illness, and were worried and upset about everything. However, over time, the therapist managed to carve out a message the parents could hear.

I remember vividly the advice the therapist gave to the mother, which the mom shared with me. I have used it countless times in helping to steady the nerves of an anxious and disappointed premed—and my own daughter. Just to really condense it here, the message was this: When your child tells you that something in their environment has caused them to experience a crisis or catastrophic results, you need to have a dual response, one internal, to yourself, and the other external, to your child.

To yourself, in the privacy of your mind, you say: *That's life. That's life.* In other words, find a quick phrase or mantra you can say to yourself where you accept what has happened: You completely and 100% accept the reality, inside yourself. You do not necessarily accept your child's version, particularly of the implications of what has happened. That's the job of a parent: You accept what has happened. You do not say to your child:

Oh, I'm sure it wasn't that bad, or you're overreacting. You're so dramatic or you tend to take things hard. You're so sensitive.

Don't lessen it. Don't even try to alleviate it. And do not agree that blame is the answer:

You are right. That person is a totally horrible person.

Instead, you allow silence, and in the silence, you just say to yourself. *That's life.* Because that thing has happened and that reaction has happened and the behavioral response has happened. You can change the future if you stay in the present, but you cannot change the past. So you just say to yourself. *That's life.* Here's a good pointer from Rachel Naomi Remen, the pediatrician and physician burnout expert, to strengthen your discipline:

> *Perhaps the most important thing we bring to another person is the silence in us, not the sort of silence that is filled with unspoken criticism or hard withdrawal. The sort of*

> *silence that is a place of refuge, of rest, of acceptance of someone as they are. We are all hungry for this other silence.*

But then, what do you say to your child who is looking to you for sympathy and validation?

You say to your child: *That sucks.* Or if you find that vulgar, you could say: *That stinks.* No more elaboration is needed. To yourself you say: *That's life.* To your child you say: *That sucks.*

And basically, that's how you show up for them without acting on the compulsion parents sometimes feel that they have to fix everything. Parent as fixer is a mirage of modern life. If you pose as a fixer, in the end, they may, and probably will, just argue with you about all the mistakes you made trying to fix things.

Gina spent a year preparing to take the MCAT. She had finished all the course prerequisites after college, including one that was hard to find. She moved from Philadelphia to a little remote town in northern Wisconsin for a summer so she could take this particular course in the only place she could find it. After that, she returned home, took her MCAT after a sleepless, anxious night, and when she saw her score, 35 long days later, she instantly knew it was not good enough. She called me as soon as she got the score. She went home to her family's house and she was crying and crying and crying.

A little later, she called back, strong and composed, and she said, *my mom has found a solution. She is taking me out for ice cream. So everything is going to feel better soon.* What Gina's mom said was, in effect: *That sucks: let's go out for ice cream. Let's go, let's go do something mildly satisfying and enjoy. Enjoy, while you get through this, with me alongside for company.* So after ice cream with her mom, Gina was able to realize that what she would prefer to do was to withdraw from that cycle and to retake the exam. Gina's mother innately sensed that the only thing she could do was to let Gina's confidence naturally rebound. By engaging in an ordinary diversion, it helped Gina to accept the temporary obstacles, to ease letting go of them.

The obstacles usually take the form of self-criticism. When a score, grade or authority's feedback is not good, the applicant can begin to rationalize and justify self-criticism, obsessively generating solutions and fixes as a defense against despair. A parent who resists offering solutions and fixes is one who models resilience. *You can handle this. You can still become a physician, even though something negative has happened.* When the despair has abated, you can say something like: *I have faith that you will know how to handle this.* The first person who pulls together their confidence could be you, actually, modeling strength.

After plenty of more time studying and fruitfully addressing her anxiety, Gina retook the MCAT, and did much better. She gained admission to six medical schools, then withdrew from her remaining interview dates and her other applications. Remarkable how not trying to fix things—along with a little ice cream outing—can pave the way to recovery.

Here are some other perfectly natural responses to negative stressors that you should not use. As I said earlier, do not complain of and/or blame other people or institutions. Second, do not try to produce a solution or fix, or introduce your own idea of a mindset change: another way of thinking or another way of looking at it, and why the applicant should adopt your new way. That mindset change is for them to come up with. It is not the time, and in fact, the time rarely comes when working with a premed on their application cycle to say: *This is not the end of the world.* Perspective comes later.

Finally, don't reward perfectionism. Even if you have seen it repeatedly in your child's life course, even if they got it from your own perfectionism, always try to adopt a bemused shrug of puzzled-ness when you see the post-perfection, crushed ego, crop up at a time when perfect is just simply not what's going on.

Of all the things you should not say, what you should never say is that it is okay with you if they do not become a physician. That is the all-time, cardinal no-no. *You know, honey, you really don't have to be a doctor, you have so many qualities that do not require standardized testing. There are so many ways you can help people. There are so many ways that you can, you know, live large in the world. You just don't have to go through this honey. Believe me, I love you, without it. I love you, if you don't ever become a doctor.* A comment like that makes them absolutely, insanely furious. If you want to see a tempest in a teapot in your own living room, just try saying that at the wrong time.

Of course there are exceptions to this directive. If they ask you if you are okay with them changing career plans, of course you would say it's okay. Anytime you are asked directly by your child to release them from whatever they perceive to be your expectations, go for it. The point is that parents signal a wavering of confidence when they talk up alternative careers and that usually just makes things harder to bear and harder to bounce back from.

You may ask, when **is** the time to provide perspective? Let's just be systematic here. We covered the main things that you should never say, and now we will cover why as a parent, you need to regain your own confidence as your child is regaining their confidence. You need to check in with yourself. Do you feel as devastated about this setback as your child does? Well then, you're identifying too much with your child and their life and you need to gain some perspective on your own. Not through talking to them, but by processing it inside yourself or talking to a friend, spouse, or even a professional. Because by definition, you should not feel as badly as they do about their setbacks. Because they need you to throw the lifeline, not to drown with them.

So you need to be confident and that means that you need to ask yourself: *Do I have faith that Julie is still going to be able to become a doctor?* And if your honest answer is no, then you need to just sit there and say to her, again: *That sucks. What can I do to temporarily divert your attention from this horrible moment?*

But if the answer is yes, then the thing to do is to reach over when they emerge from self-absorption and are looking at you and you feel you have their attention. Don't demand or seize their attention. Don't say: *Look at me! I need to tell you something really important!* Not like that, but rather, you just wait. While you are waiting, you show up as a present being in their life. You just wait attentively, and then when you see that they are with you, you say: *I have complete faith that if you want to become a doctor, you will become a doctor.* Don't say it until you mean it, because your child has observed you for at least 20 years, sometimes much longer, and they know when you're faking it.

Really Having Faith, Yourself

If you fake it, they will know you're faking it, and the best outcome you could hope for is for them to be glad that they have a nice mommy or daddy who's willing to fake it to help them, but it won't really inject or inoculate their spirit with: *I can do this. I'm going to still be able to do this.* Because it has to be true. It has to really be true. You have to feel it inside your bones, at the level of spirit.

Spiritual growth and development, and living out of the messages of your spirit are essential elements of being good company on the journey to medical school and to a career in medicine. Everyone you may have seen in person or on TV; tele-evangelists, or New Age gurus, preachers and rabbis, all know how to say great and inspiring words, but we have all had the experience of being, at best, completely unmoved by them and, at worst, finding them laughable or pathetic. They don't touch your spirit when you feel like they're phony or fake. We have all had that experience, and seen funny movies depicting religion-peddling shysters who use religious revival movements in order to enrich their fur-lined pockets.

You can see right through it and so don't think your child can't see right through it. You need to cultivate your own faith during this process, and the best way I know to do that is for you to declare your faith in your child's ability to handle anything. Ancient rituals and practices exist to help people submerge their own will to a higher good. Spoken affirmations, prayers, even chants can help sustain and strengthen the confidence muscle. You can simply write a sentence that really appeals to you about your faith in your child, and you can say it every morning, an affirmation of your love and your confidence in your child. Put it on an index card and carry it around with you. Say it all the time, sending your good intentions in their direction on a spiritual plane, which may work better than through a text message. Metta or loving kindness meditations also help both you and your child:

May you be safe. May you be free from suffering. May you be at peace. May you be happy. (May you get a different organic chemistry lab instructor next semester).

Timing is very important because you don't just want to slather your premed with affirmations—*I believe in you. I think you're good and you're going to make it*—all the time because then they will become habituated to your message and they will no longer really hear it for the impact that it has. Also, praising qualities like intelligence, or other character traits does not boost confidence because innate characteristics/talents are not something they can change. Instead, thank them and show respect for actions like hard work, grit, perseverance, strengths that your premed has control over and can strengthen. You don't have to be self-confident yourself—although it certainly helps—in order to have confidence in your child.

It's really important that you recognize mutual confidence as one of the most emotionally intimate parts of your relationship that you may ever have with your child. We forget about the intimacy of that because when you raise a child who has what it takes to become a doctor, who has that kind of discipline, tenacity, self control, management of desire, when you have someone that awesome and you get to have them as your child, you cannot help but feel really proud of them.

Naturally, you want to share their story with the people in your family and your friends, and even people who aren't your friends, such as business associates. A successful young adult child is just such a badge to wear as a parent. And you have to recognize that the badge that you wear and the pride that you put out into the world is very, very different from the confidence that you share directly with your child. Frankly, many children feel that they get that spiritual nourishment, that deep confidence reboot from their grandparents in a way that they don't get it from their parents, because it's a simpler relationship. The grandparents are grateful that the grandchild is in their life and wants to talk to them and have a relationship with them. And out of that deep gratitude, which is not taken for granted, as it can be with a parent, a grandparent can often say just the right thing at the right time. Their life is less cluttered. They may brag to their friends about your premed, but when they're with them, they are just genuinely curious about them and grateful that they want to share. Gratitude is another important thing to bring to the parent/young adult relationship.

A regular meditation practice can be so valuable for both you and your premed. Meditation can also help to relieve anxiety. Sometimes as parents we care so much about our child's hopes and dreams that we become more attached to them then they are, and can actually become terrified of what happens if they don't achieve them. Meditation can help lessen that anxiety, which is all too transmissible in intimate relationships and may prove inevitably detrimental to our child, even to the point of undermining their sense that we have confidence in them. Meditation can be quick too, as quick as brushing your teeth in the morning. And while it is one more daily thing to do, it allows you to really clarify some false beliefs you might be carrying around with you.

Addressing Overconfidence

I have heard from parents that they worry about the opposite problem with confidence. What if I feel my child is too confident or too full of themselves? Is that a problem that I caused, or their problem, or what can be done about it? I remember an orientation meeting with the parents of one of my applicants, Mr. Jones. We were talking over video. The dad was very matter of fact about his son's accomplishments, as well as what the dad saw as Bill's failings, like he did not get into the college where they really wanted him to go, competitively selective, but close to home. Bill's mother was lighthearted, jovial and happy, describing Bill's many lovely interpersonal qualities. It almost felt like she was trying to sell him to me.

When she knew that the sale was made, and everybody was feeling comfortable, she leaned into the laptop camera and she said: *There is one thing he needs to work on. He is terribly arrogant. It's all my fault. I read all these American parenting books when I immigrated here about how to parent a child in America because I felt like I had no idea. I had never been a parent—or an American. So I read these books, and they basically told me: Let your child follow his bliss and never reprimand him. Let him become who he is and always always tell him how great he is. Always compliment your child and praise his behavior. And so I let him follow his bliss, and now we have this incredibly accomplished kid who just thinks he's God.* The parents were hopeful that I, as the premed advisor, could help with that before he went on interviews. He is now a happy medical student at the school of his dreams, ten minutes from their home.

When your child seems overconfident, it might stem from just receiving too many empty compliments from their family, resulting in someone who has not really been disciplined by life. That's overconfidence, which is not, if you recall our early definition of confidence: coming together in faith. That is putting on a mask bearing an idealized self image, one that the premed feels he is absolutely expected to show at all times. He puts on a mask to the world that says: *You know what? I'm great. I'm unimpeachable. I can do anything.* This makes other people feel belittled and demeaned, which generates a lot of negativity around the person. People take an instant dislike to arrogant premeds.

Another thing that the mask of arrogance generates is the sense, among others, that they are not really seeing the person behind that posture. Often, experienced interviewers who are used to vetting other people, upon encountering an overconfident applicant, harbor an inner sense that the applicant is hiding something. They deduce that the applicant is actually afraid to show their true self. They extrapolate to envisioning that person as a doctor covering a hospital ward, who has been working and awake for 18 hours, puts the wrong medicine in the wrong vein and suddenly realizes their mistake. That person has to have the deep, deep confidence in themselves to go run and ask a nurse to help them. But a person who is overconfident is likely to just hope silently to God that the patient doesn't die while they try to cover up the error. Humility and confidence go together; arrogance does not coexist with humility. It is more likely to coexist with shame.

Humility is not shame and confidence is not arrogance. You might even think of these important aspects of character as being on a particular spectrum, like a seesaw, where confidence and humility need to be poised with respect to each other, like the iconic scale of justice. Confidence and humility are what medical schools want to see. Overconfidence and shame don't have any place in a doctor's professional life because the stakes are so high when they do make mistakes. They need to be able to admit their mistakes and still feel okay about themselves. To learn more about this, you can read about the concepts of growth mindset and grit, terms offered by Carol Dweck and Angela Duckworth respectively. A growth mindset incorporates confidence and humility because the person with that mindset is aware that they are capable of improvement, even when they have made a terrible mistake or one of their most shameful weaknesses is on display for all to see. The awareness that they are capable is their confidence. The awareness that there is room for improvement is their humility. Someone who exercises their growth mindset develops grit, which will sustain them through the life and death throes of a life in medicine.

I would characterize Bill, whose mother worried about his surplus of confidence, as facing a different problem with his parents. In this case, a person comes from a background that is essentially strikingly different from medicine, such as growing up with hedge fund investor parents or a father who pours concrete driveways as a sole proprietor. Bill began to sound arrogant explaining everything about getting into medical school to his parents. If you're in a profession like hedge funds or concrete construction, you've mastered your trade, so you're used to knowing everything when you show up at work, and you're used to showing up strong and confident. You come to your child armed with that essence of confident mastery, but you actually know nothing about how to get into medical school, or what it is to be a doctor. You know as little about it as any toddler coming to the rescue with a Fisher Price doctor kit knows about it.

You know nothing. So your applicant has to teach you everything. If you're really psyched to learn, you traverse the internet, trying to learn new things. If you capture all these little tidbits and myths that you find interesting, then you may become, in some sense, a well-educated, maybe even a well-informed person, but you still won't know enough about it. That's why I wrote this book, to give you an authoritative education in medical school admissions.

If your medical school aspirant takes on the role of teaching you as each next step veers over the horizon, followed by them telling you what they need, then your relative ignorance and their relative knowledge about these things can take on a certain unfavorable tinge. They may create the aura that they know more than you do—about everything. And they can then take that inflated sense of themselves out into the world. It's a kind of false bravado. It's false because, in the end, you are an expert on who they are. You don't need to remind them, but you need to know inside yourself, that you stand as an expert. You are an expert on your own young doctor to be, and their calling, which is so much more important—at the beginning, in the middle, and assuredly at the end of this process—than the details of how people gain admission into medical school.

These kids can experience a specific form of impostor syndrome, what I call the "stranger in paradise," where medical school is paradise and the premed dream is to gain the keys to paradise, but they're a stranger there. They often find reasons to feel like they are strangers. For example, they compare themselves to their friends. If their friends have siblings who are medical students or parents who are doctors, those premeds are the "insiders." If most of the people they know have more family resources of any kind, more social capital in their connections and ability to network, or seem smarter or more competent or charismatic, those people are on the "insider" track for medical school.

Because your aspirant cannot qualify through their self-defined, self-othering, stringent selection criteria as an insider, they conclude that they are an outsider. Once they identify in this way, their tendency, if they've been brought up by you to believe that they're very special and that no one like them has ever emerged into the world, then they tend to try to carry that "I am special" quality into the medical school admissions environment, which gives us a person with this message: *I am a very special outsider.* Surely you have seen this in politicians. Unfortunately, when you get up close to a person shouldering this identity baggage, well… they end up seeming kind of arrogant to other people.

This is an equal opportunity kind of arrogance. When a child grows up in a family where the means to economic security feels uncertain or complex, they can emerge conditioned to show a false bravado regarding their own path. This most commonly appears in students from low-income families or inversely, students from wealthy families who have made their fortune in high-risk ventures, such as serial entrepreneurial forays or hedge fund management. First generation, low income (FGLI) students can find it hard to connect the dots to explain how they rose out of their modest surroundings with often amorphous (even if they were very high) expectations, to get to the door of something as universally exalted as medical school. What looks like arrogance is more often rooted in what I would call an "identity risk." When a premed is the first in a successful family to attempt to become a physician, they and their nuclear family may feel and communicate that they are taking a risk, perhaps an unnecessary leap into the unknown. Therefore, the premed compensates for their family's lack of confidence (the identity risk) by a show of false confidence (which can be misperceived as arrogance).

I think this is because it's actually very weird to contemplate the roots of your own success, when you are on the one hand an ambitious kid who identifies strongly with their goal to become a doctor, and yet who can never really describe to others, or even to themselves, what specifically their parents actually do at work every day that made them financially comfortable. In the stumbling blocks they face in their pursuit of a career in medicine, ironically, FGLI kids can have much in common with the offspring of Silicon Valley venture capitalists. Both know that their families are in somewhat precarious positions economically, both long for a secure and stable career, and are willing to work hard to achieve it.

Sometimes people hire premed advisors to be a triangulating vector for the family. The advisor is appointed to be able to say things to the applicant that the parent can't really say with any authority. An advisor could easily, in the container of advising, point out to the applicant that they seem arrogant. *I know you're not. But you are coming off as full of yourself right now. That is not how you want to show up in your interviews.* An advisor like me may ask permission to tell the applicant every moment when I see that overconfidence mask showing up. Naturally, I want the applicant to understand that when I get that feeling, they should take it as just one person's impression, which is not the same as the world judging them, or a reflection of who they are at their core.

As a parent, if you feel that your premed is overconfident, it's hard to tell them that directly with any hope of effectiveness. When you tell your child that they're coming off as overconfident or arrogant, they almost always assume that it's a function of the kind of relationship you have with them as opposed to how they are in the world.

One of the very tricky parts of parenting is that there are two ways of regarding your child that are so different, but so infinitely close to each other, and they can create such different people. Way 1 is to say that *because I love you, my child, unconditionally, so does the world.* Way 2 is to say that, *even though I love you, my child, unconditionally, the world will not.*

The simple truth is that you unconditionally accept your child. I've had friends whose kids have started doing drugs at an early age, who have been absolutely unable to get out of that culture, have become addicts, have gone to jail, have killed a person when they were driving in an intoxicated state. These kids have done horrible things in their lives and my friends, their parents, still love their child, no matter what. They will mortgage their home to hire lawyers to fight for them, they will still visit them in jail, and they'll still tell others what good people their children are. You just love your child unconditionally. You see the good through any bad behavior. While you may do your level best to love your spouse and everyone else without conditions, with your child, you simply can't help but love them without conditions. You just do.

When you love someone unconditionally, the best gift you can give is to let them know that such love is possible, but at the same time, to break the news that the world around them does not always love unconditionally. *You know I do, but the world does not love you unconditionally.* There is a difference here and we should not try to convince any of our children through repetition that they are so special, all the time. Because when a child believes in the idea that they're special, then they often feel like they have to maintain that "I'm specialness" everywhere. They take that belief to mean that the rational rules of order in place at school and in the workplace do not necessarily apply to them, such as when they claim that they need an extension on homework. *I'm special, you know, I'm just a little tired tonight. I can't really stay up and finish it. So would you give me an extension without penalty?* Well…no. You're just like everybody else. Specialness is akin to separateness. Separateness sets us apart from others, whereas being normal (or being humble) connects us to all humanity, which is what we want our premeds to do in their interviews, with their classmates, and for our future doctors to be able to do.

The key understanding of these two things that are so very close to each other is the message: *while I love you unconditionally, the really important thing is for you to love yourself unconditionally, to the degree that you don't need to feel that you're more important than anyone else to get where you want to go. You don't have to be better or worse than anyone else to have your impact in medicine.* This step is not easy for any parent; it's both essential and elusive when you "give them away" to the world. One thing that makes it harder to accomplish is if you have not learned this yourself, about yourself. If you have not learned to love yourself unconditionally, it will be harder to convince your child to make this step. Sometimes your own conditional self-love, your transparent self-criticism makes it hard for them to leap into radical self-acceptance. They don't want to go beyond where you have been. It's uncomfortable. You need to do some work on yourself if you are giving this message: *You are worthy of unconditional love; I am not.*

Arrogance stems not just from confidence issues but from self-absorption. Most people I have known who are on the journey to and through medicine, think mostly about the people they want to serve. It can help the person who is leaning towards under- or over- confidence when you simply remind them that they are on a mission to become a doctor. Ask them what they feel passionate about bringing to others, to the world, at any personal cost. When they focus on their mission, and the specifics of that mission, the reasons they want to become a doctor, what they want to do for the world, it pulls the focus away from themselves and, therefore their authentic confidence just shows, and it transmits. My focus is on others and the traits they possess to realize that mission in the world, despite the obstacles. It is hard to sustain self-consciousness when focusing on others.

The application process forces premeds out of this mindset because all the essays and interviews are about their attributes and accomplishments. When they think about themselves and whether they would be a good doctor, they can feel small. But when they think of their life mission, and the contribution the world needs them to make, they just get moving toward that.

Faith traditions preach that there is a source of unconditional love that passes amongst us at all times. It is our job not to block it, and to maintain our awareness of it, to be vessels and transmitters of that unremitting, universal, unconditional love. You don't need religion to acknowledge the truth of this. You need to be able to winnow what is real from what is fantasy, what is true from what is untrue. When you work at seeing and knowing that, in your inner life and your outer life, you become the best parent ever.

These steps you take now will nourish your spirit and your premed's spirit. When she sees you as a person who truly and unconditionally loves her and supports her lifepath, she will be far less likely to be engulfed in medical school and lose touch with you. When he is so occupied and his time subsumed, he will still find time to check in with you to seek that reconnection with what really matters. Your own spiritual discovery will light his own path to truth.

To be good company on the journey that your child takes to medical school will enrich and bolster your relationship as long as you are on this Earth together, and even beyond, in the world of beautiful memories.

3 Faith and the Path to Medicine

> *...The ultimate touchstone of friendship is not improvement, neither of the other nor of the self; the ultimate touchstone is witness, the privilege of having been seen by someone and the equal privilege of being granted the sight of the essence of another, to have walked with them and to have believed in them, and sometimes just to have accompanied them for however brief a span, on a journey impossible to accomplish alone.*
>
> ~David Whyte

I have worked with many applicants who have been raised in Modern Orthodox Jewish homes. The first of these, Maryam, wanted to write her personal statement about teaching reading to young children at a local elementary school. While some advisors might consider this topic as pretty conventional and commonplace, to Maryam, it had been transformational, and that is why it was the best experience for her to develop into a personal statement. I asked her if there were any Jewish principles that she felt she brought to her teaching. Maryam responded: "Is that allowed? Are you allowed to talk about religion and faith in a personal statement?" Honestly, I was so unprepared for her question that I did not have a response that I could be certain was true for me, for her, but most important, for admissions committees. I knew Albert Einstein College of Medicine, at the time owned by Yeshiva University, would be okay with it, but what about a school that did not get many Jewish applicants or that branded itself with a western, science-based, secular vision for medical education?

I remember taking Maryam's question to a conference where admissions directors were meeting with medical school admissions advisors. And their answer was a resounding affirmative: *We love to hear about applicants' religious faith. We love to hear about their spiritual life. We just don't want to hear that they think that everyone else should join their faith and that they're going to come to medical school and convert everybody.*

A person who shies away from rooting his identity in the faith that is so precious to him may not fully express his authentic narrative, as he could and should, throughout the admissions process. A sincere effort to express one's faith to one's academic community so that others might freely learn or even choose to embrace it themselves is actually considered a virtue of the applicant.

On the other end of the declaration of faith spectrum is a person who sincerely believes it is her responsibility to proselytize to her classmates. The definition of proselytism I use here refers to an effort to convert another person, while not truly witnessing and respecting the prospective convert's own spiritual inner life. Any words or action perceived by the "convertee" as a pressure strategy directly undermines a value that admissions committees cherish: cultural humility.

Unfortunately, the premed myth that one should not give credit to a religious tenet for one's humanitarian identity because it is evangelical or proselytizing still needs to be shattered. And the way to do that is for your offspring to write about how their faith and their religion have prepared them to spend their life in a career where life and death are part of everyday deliberation.

Medical school aspirants are conditioned to understand science by their undergraduate education. They glean in their science coursework a distinctive focus on what science actually is: a methodological approach to understanding nature. Yet some science professors, in their genuine intention to teach their students to separate internet babble from evidence-based knowledge, may box learners into an utterly false dichotomy between science and faith. The people who are often most affected are those who are deeply spiritual *and* religious, as they set to work writing their medical school applications.

Spirituality and religiosity are also often set into a false dichotomy by the faith-based support networks provided by universities. You will often hear a college sophomore claiming that she is not, or is "no longer" religious, but she is spiritual. Thus to identify as religious is to run the risk of being branded, in some sense, feeble-minded. The admissions committee's concern about a medical student proselytizing their faith is trivial and rarely—if ever—occurs in medical school. The acculturation that applicants experience in the university, that faith is antagonistic to mastering science, the mental conditioning that the academic community subtly drills into their hearts and minds, is a far more potent and deeply problematic issue. All too often, it causes our open-minded premeds to deliberately de-integrate their religious life, their own experience of the power and promise of faith, and cleave it away from their academic life. As they learn how to think systematically about natural phenomena through the scientific method, they increasingly compartmentalize what they see and sense, know and intuit, from their professor's concept of scientific evidence as providing the more real truth of how nature works. This bodes ill for their mental health and even bodes ill for science and medicine.

Maryam taught me about Tikkun Olam in her personal statement, once she became convinced that she could fully share who she is in that document. Tikkun Olam, a Jewish tenet, mandates that making the world a better place is a requirement for human conduct. It is essential to living a life grounded in faith. This is just one of many important and well-developed concepts of virtue that are rooted in the moral tenets of the Jewish tradition.

Applicants need the language of faith-based traditions to express these virtues in their writing. They worry, and you might also, that their audience will not appreciate their words. Applicants may claim that the medical school admissions reader is no different from their undergraduate science lecturers, who push the idea that the scientific construct is a value at the top of the hierarchy of human values. Their teachers have pushed this concept of science as being The Truth, that grows out of double blind, randomized controlled studies. The science journals they read, if they are so lucky to be exposed to them in their undergraduate studies, train a laser focus on peer review. Peer review would never allow anything to be published that did not emerge from a well-constructed research study. Thus, our premeds conclude, only science is worth writing about and faith is meritless in considering publication in a science journal.

This overemphasis on a reductionist view of science facilitates their achievement in their science classes; that's the benefit of it. The downside is that it can make our future doctors feel like religion and talking about religion makes them look cognitively inferior or as having a second-rate mind. This is a really powerful lever in suppressing students' religious discovery and practice. Even more important, the conditioning that cleaves science from faith teaches our young doctors-to-be to suppress their spirituality. And by spirituality, I mean, the sense they have that they're connected to something both inside them and flowing through and out of them, a true force of nature that is both unique and universal at the same time. The spirit you love that you see in them is what I am talking about.

They need us to remind them that the original insight the scientist had began as an act of faith rooted in the alignment of mind, heart and spirit: their received wisdom. This led to the hypothesis that was tested and confirmed in the published article, which then became accepted as fact. A scientist is a powerful practitioner of Tikkun Olam—to heal the world—when she simply expresses how her scientific understanding has grown from her faith and direct observation of nature. As noted astronomer Carl Sagan wrote: *Science is not only compatible with spirituality; it is a profound source of spirituality.*

In fact, all scientists have faith in the unseen. That's why they spend their lives creating informed hypotheses and testing things out to see if they can validate them—because they think that something is true, which no one yet knows for sure is true. That part of science is rarely shared with applicants—and it needs to be. If all the premed applicant has is you, a parent, to share it, then you should invite it regularly, and conduct guided discussions with them where they can sort out the myth of a dichotomy between faith/spirituality and science.

If you raised your child in a very religiously observant home, you have probably had plenty of opportunities to observe the ways in which the tenets of your shared religion have shown up in the personality and spirit of your offspring. It's worth your time to sit down and for you to write about that so that you can share it with your offspring when they are most in need of hearing it. For example, if you have a child who is clearly energized—as opposed to drained or dispirited—by the service that she's doing in a clinical setting for underserved patients, you might comment on that somewhat paradoxical observation. *It's such hard work; why aren't you tired?* You could say the reason that your premed has a lot of energy for that work probably comes from the deep-seated generosity that they were born with that you have seen show up in many places throughout their life.

Many applicants write about how, when they were young, their parents took them to places like soup kitchens and put an apron on them and the whole family, as they worked together one shift a week or one shift every couple of weeks. And parents who do that with their children instill in them a sense of *this is part of our daily life, to give to others,* which is also a central tenet of most religious practice, precisely because it is an outward manifestation of their inner spirituality.

To be a person for others, a Jesuit vow, is fundamental to becoming a mentally healthy physician. You must gain energy from the particular service you provide as a doctor to be regenerated each day by your work. That's just true. But being a person for others is just one aspect of developing a spiritual focus to one's career in medicine. In addition to the things that people do for each other, one of the most critical reasons to be connected to your spirit is because it keeps you whole, while life and the world buffet you around. By whole, I mean that it is much harder to break a person who is deeply and immediately connected to their spirit, because when one is connected, they can more easily and readily sift what matters from what doesn't matter, even in a crisis or catastrophic situation.

You may be actually afraid that if you told your applicant, *your problem is you need to be more religious or you need to come to church with me,* that they might resist that. Or they might fight you and say, *that's not the answer to my suffering or unease.* You would both be right, but right and wrong do not matter when we are talking about nurturing the muscle of spirit in the people we love. Many young adults resist regular attendance at traditional places of worship, not only as a way of asserting their own control over their time, but also as a way of questioning the meaning of it all. Do not see this as a reason for alarm on your part. Better to see it as a way that the aspirant can use to get in touch with the deeper meanings of the religion that they've been raised in.

After all, attendance at worship functions represents the community part of the religion. People look out for each other and treat each other with kindness and niceties to feel like they have fellowship and community with each other. All that communing grew out of something that everyone assumes that each other has, which is a deep personal relationship to their own spirit. And sometimes people will opt out of church because they need to go into a seeking phase. They have lost the signal due to the noise, lost their reception of the spiritual transmission that fuels communal worship.

I think a more fruitful place to start is to acknowledge that you, as a parent, need to make an effort to see your adult child, maybe for the first time. The love you have for them allows you to see them, but you need to let go of the conditions that parenting puts on children so you can establish what Buddhists call "right relationship." Through one necessity at a time, you may have wedged your unconditional love for your child into a set of conditions by which they must earn your love.

If you don't pick up your shoes, and put them away, you're not going to get dessert tonight. Or maybe you put things very positively rather than punitively: *When you put away your shoes, you make me happy.* You've been talking like that since your children were old enough to put away their shoes, hopefully, and now you have to dissolve the conditionality because spirituality simply does not flourish in an atmosphere of conditionality. You need to get on the road back to expressing the truly unconditional love you have for your medical school aspirant, which is not easy.

You could start by simply stating that you both need to abandon the idea that they need to earn your acceptance or, by extension, your love through their actions, accomplishments or achievements. You could gently point out that you know their love for you has never been conditioned in this way, and that you had to use conditioning to get them to adopt certain habits related to hygiene, harmonious living with others and self-care throughout their childhood. Tell them that they are autonomous beings now, and you are here to guide, help and bear witness without rewards and punishments, including judgments. You do reserve the right to laud their high points to family members and even confide your despair in their setbacks to your own friends, however! This is a sacred oath of the high privilege of parenting a young adult, and if you cannot in all honesty do this, you need to do some inner work yourself to become the parent you want to be, a facilitator of the bumpy road to true, autonomous, independent adult life.

4 View into the Admissions Office

Nearly every medical doctor has an admissions cycle in her rearview mirror. Many will tell you that it was the hardest period of their lives. Harder than the pedagogical fire hose of the first 18-24 months of medical school, harder than residency 24-hour on-call months, harder than the first month of infant parenting. That's a lot of stuff to be harder than. The trials of the admission cycle leave an indelible impression, which helps to explain why everybody who is still hanging around in academic medicine years after that fraught period of getting into medical school has more than a passing interest in the local medical school's admissions process.

Priorities in the Admissions Office

The medical school administration cares about who is matriculating at their medical school for many reasons. These include reputation, which is quantified by ratings based on numerical reductions, the most obscene (by general consensus of all stakeholders) being the average MCAT/GPA that factors into US News & World Report. Everyone on the clinical faculty cares about the intellectual and human characteristics of the medical student cohort they will be instructing. Everyone in the institutional development fundraising group cares about the potential career impacts of the students the school is training. The farther the graduates go, the friendlier they tend to be to the medical school that trained them...with considerations that may include preferential treatment at residency selection when they become residency directors, and financial gifts to the school earned from lucrative careers that provide ample discretionary philanthropy.

The Student Affairs people care about bringing in enough strong, resilient, well-adjusted, altruistic and culturally inclusive students to help keep the culture positive. They care that people with histories of mental illness or hidden disabilities know how and when to get the support they need to manage the rigors of medical school. The Diversity Affairs office is vested in recruiting and supporting a critical mass of diversity along all dimensions so no one feels alone, marginalized, different or misunderstood. In addition, a truly diverse class, like a diverse investor portfolio, leads to a stronger graduating class with eclectic backgrounds, interests and strengths. A building block of true diversity means having some class members who relate to each other's particular set of identity or socioeconomically rooted struggles. The alumni who are giving back of their time and material success want to see medical students whom they can relate to and mentor with ease.

When the admissions office tries to take all this into consideration, you need to understand that politics and power hierarchies do come into play. People in power at centers of medical education, people in the "C-Suite" (CEO, COO, CIO and CFO) and Trustees, for example, have to deal with such an array of competing factions, stakeholders and high-impact decision making on a daily basis, it's natural that they wish they could have a little clout in admissions. Helping a premed gain a leg up can seem like a fringe benefit, a job perk.

Application Review

Consider the structure of the admissions office. When the applications flow in, lower level administrators check them for completeness. Many, many applications are never completed. Screening for interviews often starts with a computer-based applicant-sorting algorithm that is quantitative in nature, which is why the MCAT/GPA metrics may figure largely into this process. They are simply numbers, easy to compute. While applicants are generally not rejected outright as a result of that algorithm-based sorting process, they are usually consigned to virtual piles that differentiate them by level of admissions selection potential. For example, people with identities of great recruiting interest who have somewhat lower metrics may be separated from others for a second look, whereas applications from others with those lower metrics who do not have these "identities of interest" may be deposited into a lower priority and deeper pile. Due to the semi-automated sorting process, applicants who are sorted out must wait for further screening. This sorted-out applicant who must wait for further screening is the kind of applicant who benefits most immediately from an outside advocate, whose work we will discuss later. Screening is done by many people and the best admissions offices have effective, enforced training for reviewers.

Unfortunately, many, if not most admissions offices, do not have this. The admissions office sometimes has to beg around to find volunteer readers and sometimes they have to have two readers per file, who are doing this after everything else they need to do for their day job is put away for the day. Other schools have diligently lobbied their administration for funding so they can hire the readers they need. Either the admissions office has trained, compensated, disciplined and effective readers, or they seek volunteers, and of course many combinations exist between these two poles. The best practice is to have sufficient reviewers of sufficient competence just to get through the many thousand applications they need to read. The reality can be that, given the avalanche of applications, the admissions offices at medical schools are understaffed. From the applicant point of view, the truth is: it's not easy to get a truly fair review.

Who Is In Charge?

At the head of the admissions office is almost always a Dean, usually a rising faculty member who relishes the role of admissions decision maker for all the reasons cited above, and who very frequently executes many institutional roles. These physician administrators frequently have their own clinical practices, teach in the medical school, and sometimes they also manage Student Affairs.

The Director of Admissions is a staff position. Sometimes the Director is promoted to Assistant Dean.[4] The MD who supervises the office is usually given the title of Associate Dean. The important thing to keep in mind is that one is faculty and the other is a staff position. Together, the Dean and Director manage the committee review process. First, applications are assembled and rendered complete. Then they are screened and distributed into different subgroups based on their appeal, how well they fit the attributes the school seeks, and its diversity aims. Once a group is invited to interview and has been evaluated by the interviewer, they are either admitted outright, rejected outright, or sent to committee.

The Dean relies on the Director to keep the admissions cycle running on time and to prepare the applicant reviews for admissions committee consideration. The Dean chairs the committee. I have observed admissions deliberations at a few schools wholly from the perspective of a premed advisor who was so lucky to be invited, and I have seen some significant ways that they differ. To me, the best model is one where the Dean facilitates productive and fair discussion and the Director keeps things moving.

The committee members come from as many different sectors of the medical school as possible. This includes students from year 1 through 4, residents, clinical faculty, pedagogic faculty,

---

4 Promoting the Director of Admissions to the Assistant Dean title is often a naming compliment, prompting the ordering of new business cards and little else, rendering this staff person to appear to be a faculty facsimile when they face outward to the sea of premeds who seek their attention and approval. To their colleagues in the admissions community, the new title simply means they earned their change of title, probably has the same duties but maybe got a pay raise along with it, and has been around awhile.

including PhD scientists (non-MD faculty), everybody staffing the Student Affairs office, from diversity officers, to learning specialists, to disability coordinators, to financial aid and career opportunities specialists. They all agree that they should aim to recruit a diverse range of people for the admissions committee, of different races, genders, and ages sitting around the table, from the twenty-somethings to the mid-career, mid-life employees to the aging retirees who want to give back and supply a little wisdom and history. There should be a fair and equitable staff-faculty mix. This mixture demands that a lot of busy people show up on a weeknight at 4:30 pm for hummus, carrot sticks, pita, and conversation, while maintaining their focus on each applicant under scrutiny, in turn.

The Deans are leaders who often don't express much of an opinion, but they reign in the grandstanders. Every committee has them. Here 's a conversation I witnessed at an admissions committee I was invited to sit in on once: *Should we really be giving such a high level of favor to people doing Teach for America (a two year program where people teach in underperforming schools)? There are so many of them; they are crowding out the other applicants. I move that we only give extra favor to those who do at least two consecutive terms of Teach for America. Then we can really believe that they are service-oriented.*

The Dean makes sure everyone with a considered point of view on the applicant has the chance to voice it. They diplomatically hush debate on matters like whether you need two rounds of Teach for America to get into their school.

Every institution of higher learning has a sharp break in discretionary decision making right at the gaping divide between faculty and staff. Directors face the applicants and some have considerable weight in admissions decisions, but mostly they don't. This is why it can be frustrating to appeal to a Director of Admissions who really likes your premed, respects their narrative and would like to have them at their medical school, but just can't make that happen.

Committee Decisions

All schools do admissions decision making differently, but here is a typical scenario. The committee reviews applicants after the interviewers have rated them. The interviewers present the applicant, navigating the applicant's files verbally and present their rationale for their interview ratings. After a brief conversation, either the member with the higher rating drops his rating or the lower rating person raises hers, or they agree to disagree, and in either case, the committee votes. People who received uniformly high or uniformly low ratings at interviews are generally put in the accept or reject piles without the committee's initial input. Often there are finalist meetings to go over those applicants who are in the preliminary accept pile. Usually there are more applicants in that pile than seats in the medical school, often by a factor of four. This is where it gets painful and outside advocacy can help break a tie.

At some schools, the committee keeps a tight rein on final offers; at others, the Dean has some personal discretion. Rarely does the Director have any, but they can offer timely comments and suggestions. Some Directors have been around a long time, longer than their Deans, and have earned a lot of discretion about how decisions are made. Often they can make decisions, particularly off the alternate or waitlist. The amount of discretion that the admissions officers hold is alway a tightly held secret, and they enjoy it when they can garner more. Little if any transparency lies there.

During the admissions committee meeting, the Director shovels relevant info to the Dean, who they usually sit beside in the meeting, while tracking the commentary and the final votes. Sometimes the Director speaks up with a relevant thought or point about the applicant, such as: *She was rude to the admissions staff because she got lost, arrived late and then blamed it on the administrative assistant's directions.* (Doom awaits that applicant.) Or: *Her personal statement might give you some insight into that C+ in Orgo. Do you have that in front of you?* (Wake up and read the application, Dr. Overworked!)

I personally appreciate the work of Admissions Directors and feel just a bit sorry for them. They are the face of the admissions office and they travel to fairs where they meet tons of wonderful premeds who seek their approval. They get to be the face of the medical school, to spout the storylines of opportunity and unique programs the schools have scripted for them, but they don't generally exercise all that much influence over decisions. Most of the time, the best work they can do is to stand for fairness under the pressure of other, more powerful influencers, so that makes it even harder for them to push for their own favorites. In the chapter on applicant networking, I explain how to become that favorite in the hopes that somewhere along the line the Admissions Director can get to see themselves as a facilitator of hopes and dreams, one who opens the gate to worthy young doctors. This is a far more rewarding role than that of gate closer who needs to send out rejection letters to people who made it all the way to the accept pile only to be bumped into the reject pile at the last minute, like airlines do when they oversell their seats on a flight. It's hard to derive personal satisfaction from that role and it's hard to be on the low end of the medical school political hierarchy when you have so much responsibility for such an important element of it.

Points of Networking and Advocacy

Given the context above, we now turn to networking and its natural outcome, effective advocacy in the admissions process, with some ideas of how to start and to effectively help your premed. No medical school admissions office works exactly like that depicted above, but the features I described serve as instructional vehicles for the work that lies ahead for you in terms of strategizing with your premed the most effective networking and advocacy plan for these important inflection points in the admissions cycle: before the invitation to interview, when put on hold before or after initial committee review, and after a decision puts the premed on the alternate or waitlist.

5 Using Your Social Capital: Intergenerational Networking

I am writing about networking to you, one who loves and cares for a premed, fully realizing that you may already identify in one of two camps regarding your capacity to network on behalf of your applicant. Either you feel well-connected and well-resourced, or you feel helplessly unconnected. To the former I say: *Mind the pitfalls of overworking your connections as a privileged social being—or your actions might backfire.* To the self-identified unconnected person, I say: *You have many more vectors into the world of medical school admissions than you might think.* To both, the most important news of all: *When you teach and encourage your premed to stay tuned into the shifting, evolving and expanding network that surrounds them every day, they will learn to network to great benefit.* Two initially separate and distinct networks operate in your sphere of medical school admissions, your direct network and your premed's direct network, which I will specifically address in a later chapter. As you enter the medical school admissions years, you want the networks to merge and continue to expand through your thoughtful approaches.

Before the admissions cycle, when you know your premed is going to apply, think about who you know and who they know. Get organized. Look through all the ways that we archive our connections to other people, digitally and not digitally. Leave no stone unturned. Talk things over with your premed and reach an agreement on how and when you will network.

What is the goal? To connect with someone who can ask an admissions dean or director for a closer review of your premed's candidacy or application for medical school.

The most effective advocacy during the admissions cycle is well timed. There are no ironclad rules, as each medical school is different. Generally, the review for interview season begins in July and continues through November, when it slows down, and then resumes in January. Those are the prime months. By March, things are pretty slow, if not over. November and December are iffy because of holidays and because the admissions offices are very busy just handling the process. They try to wind things up and get through some of their backlog so they can all take a little time off at the end of the year.

One suppressed, conditioned assumption about medical school admissions bears examination. Because applying to medical school is an expensive undertaking, we all agree that our premeds need financial capital, the more the better, in order to gain admission to more than one school and to schools they will love. You could go on a very nice three-week high-season luxury trip to another continent for the same price as financing your premed's medical school admissions cycle. This gambit involves so much sacrifice. But financial capital is just at the very base of what they will need. Precious few people earn all by themselves the funds they need to apply to medical school. Most are financed either through their family's investment or some form of financial assistance program offered by the medical school application services and the individual medical colleges.

But this chapter is about social capital, and here's some good news: most people can autonomously, without money, earn the social capital they will need to have the best chance possible of getting in. Social capital is built by calling on the networks you and your premed have built, while you continue to build them out. Social capital is even more important than financial capital and everyone can raise it. Consider where you have been and what connections you made in those locations. Become rich in your connections to others!

I was talking about this with my sister, Tracey, who is a business coach in Portland, Oregon. She was prompted by our conversation to go to LinkedIn, to see if she knew anyone who was associated with a medical school in any capacity. A friends' granddaughter was planning to apply to medical school. Within half a minute, Tracey was surprised to see that Melissa, one of her closest friends, has a brother who is an admissions dean at a medical school in another state. She knew Melissa's brother was a doctor, but not that he worked at a medical school. Tracey invited her two friends, who knew each other before only vaguely, out for lunch and explained the connection between the brother and the granddaughter. Voilà! The needle moves in favor of the granddaughter!

Networking During High School and College Years

Premeds are professionally oriented and they want to spend time on activities that prepare them for their medical careers and also help them get into medical school. As a parent, you can facilitate their engagement in these activities outside the iceberg of their college education. Here are some things they like and ought to be doing:

- Helping others
- Thinking about the science and quantitative subjects they study
- Being around and contributing to the work of research labs
- Learning about medicine, both in clinics and formal study
- Learning about, and becoming personally engaged with socioeconomic and healthcare issues
- Engaging in and developing their personal passions; music, arts, movement, travel, culture, relationships with family, friends and partners

- Helping to initiate, organize and sustain service, clinical, research and passion-pursuits and to pursue professional training opportunities outside of school

You can keep your eyes and ears open to help guide them to these opportunities. I suggest you keep a notebook, or even a spreadsheet, where you brainstorm these things. This is training-wheels networking for the future applicant. You know someone who knows someone who runs a cardiology lab in the medical school near you. Ask them to set up a meeting or a cup of coffee so you and your premed can talk with them about her interests in the lab and what other opportunities she can find at the school. Coffee shops in this country, if you have not noticed already, are the engine that drives connection. After graduating from Harvard, one of my applicants got a job as a barista in a coffee shop near Wall Street. She found that she learned more in her year there about connecting with and building networks, while pulling espresso shots and wiping tables within earshot of occupied tables, than she learned from four years in her Ivy League academic culture.

Networking to help your premed find a great summer or gap year job or academic year volunteer gig will help them get into medical school. It will help them to surround themselves with the people who work at these places, who can mentor them, write them letters of recommendation and help them find their way to the next gig.

Networking During the Admissions Cycle

Dr. Louis Kuchnir is a Boston-based dermatologist. Growing up as the child of academics and later earning a PhD at one institution and his MD at another, he was keenly aware of the circles that academics form in order to move into greater arenas of influence. While he loved learning, teaching, and doctoring, he turned his talents to founding a successful and growing dermatology and dermatologic surgery practice in the region surrounding Boston, Massachusetts. Wanting to nurture and give expression to his mentoring and teaching gifts, he formed a special program—probably the first of its kind—to give a year of paid intensive exposure to clinical medicine to a recruited and carefully curated cohort of premeds who wanted to spend a year or two between college and medical school outside of academia.

One of the many things his doctor assistants learn outside the clinic is how to network to have a successful medical career. He teaches them that potential influencers in one's network make a difference on the basis of two essential criteria: access and motivation. Simply put, networking can work for your premed if they have a contact who has direct access to the admissions office and when that contact is motivated to help them. I add a third element to access and motivation: timing. Just because I have access to an admissions director Ms. B, and am motivated to reach out to Ms. B to help you get into her medical school, does not mean I know when or how to reach out in the approximately two year long admissions cycle, or why my outreach will have an impact on Ms. B's own access and more important, her motivation to help me or you.

Here's an example of a well-connected family and how her networking played out. Emily was a great applicant to medical school. She had it all, great college, exceptional grades at a university known for its rigor, unmatched extracurricular leadership, innovation, legacy, a kind, humble and personable manner, wit, smarts and total commitment to medicine. She was an ideal candidate for her dream school. She did have one noteworthy deficiency in her academic record: her MCAT score was on the low side of average.

Her grandfather had served as an attending and teaching physician on the faculty of an urban medical school for his entire career and Emily dreamed of studying there under his benevolent shadow. She wanted to make him proud and for him to know she was carrying on his legacy. Her grandfather was a beloved icon at the school. Sharp of mind and body, he was still working and practicing. Emily's father was Counsel to the President of the Board of Trustees at the same medical school. Emily grew up in the city where this medical school operated. The school was in the mid-selective range and known for holistic admissions, which meant the MCAT/GPA metric was slightly less important for this school than others, and it was known to favor applicants who appreciated its mission and really wanted to go there.

Emily applied broadly, leaving nothing to chance due to her MCAT score. She was subsequently invited to interview at several schools in her state but none outside, likely due to the MCAT screening her out, and was admitted outright to two schools. At her dream school, where her network converged and her family had done strategic reaching out and asking for her to be given a VIP chance, she was interviewed. She had a positive, even exhilarating interview day and her interviewers gave her very promising and positive feedback. A month later, her decision arrived by email: waitlisted. Months later, late in the cycle, Emily was offered acceptance off the waitlist and she became a very happy and self-realized medical student at her dream school. She sent me a photo of her grandpa helping her into her white coat at the college's ceremony installing its newest students. Tears rose when I saw that.

Many onlookers would have predicted that Emily would have an early interview and acceptance. Why didn't this happen? Medical schools may open doors for people with strong social capital, but they do not invite people over the threshold if they don't do the work to show they belong there on their own merits.

The admissions committee certainly gotten the memo that Emily had VIP connections. They certainly saw in reviewing her file that she was an applicant at the level of excellence they seek to populate their class. But they also knew that her MCAT typically, even along with everything else that was so great, would land an applicant on the alternate list. So they put her there, to be fair, and as she continued to write them, advocating for herself without breathing a mention of her sources of external influence, as she made the case for herself, she inched ever higher on the list of people who would likely be accepted once a seat opened. From the medical school committee perspective, they know from the outset that it's very likely that they will matriculate Emily. If they chose outright and early on to admit another applicant who was not so well-connected as Emily, but equivalently suitable and great, that other applicant, if they were on the fence, might be more likely to matriculate at their school, increasing their all-important yield, due to the compliment of being accepted outright. They probably knew Emily would wait for them.

What's our takeaway? Networking helps get attention, but it doesn't score the seat. Sometimes it even pushes the applicant into a certain pigeonhole. Emily's nearly ideal sphere of influence didn't backfire in its attempts, as it well could have, but it was still up to her to prove her mettle.

Let's look at an applicant whose father died when she was six, and whose mother raised the three children she was left with: 6, 3 and 18 months at the time, all by herself. When Liza applied to medical school, her mom worked as a mid-level administrator for a nanny-placement agency. Just like Emily, Liza had everything going for her but one insufficient MCAT subscore. She took it twice and got the same subscore. She decided to apply and hope for the best. The cycle started out slow. Nothing happened for months. Liza's mother decided to call a doctor who had used the agency's services in hiring a nanny and had been grateful to her for her assistance at that time. She craved advice on how to help Liza. This was the only doctor she knew that wasn't her or her children's doctor. Turns out the doctor was now a faculty member at a medical school where Liza had applied!

Liza's mother asked the doctor to speak with her daughter about the school and the doctor agreed. Liza wrote to the doctor asking for the meeting three separate times, as another month went by, before she got a reply. The meeting was set, and Liza and I prepared for it as if it were a choreographed production: costume, script, locale, follow up scenarios. We set the goal: increase the doctor's motivation to gain access to someone on the admissions committee to encourage the admissions office to give Liza an interview. Liza's meeting with the doctor went according to plan and then Liza proceeded to regularly and gently inquire if the doctor had discerned and spoken to someone on the admissions committee. The tact and good energy communication this kind of campaign takes rarely comes naturally. Liza took it on as professional development training and we spent a lot of time and energy premeditating each step and debating different forms of communication: hand written note, email, sent at what time of day and what time of week, or phone call?

The indirect gain of this approach is that it increased Liza's confidence and reminded her of how much the goal of becoming a physician—not just a medical student—mattered to her and that all this extra work would be worth it in the end. This story has a happy ending too. Liza had her interview and was accepted at the medical school. By the time that happened, Liza had extended her newly polished networking skills, developing new contacts at expanded venues, and was dispatching them at many other schools, where she also interviewed and was accepted. In the end, she held several acceptances and was able to choose her favorite, where she is flourishing.

At the beginning of the cycle, when Liza was faced with the unfortunate MCAT subscore, I reached out to a colleague who is a dean, the longstanding faculty chair of his school's admissions committee. I asked him to review her carefully and look beyond the MCAT subscore. He wrote back that while he appreciated her qualities, the subscore was just too low for their consideration. In this case, my own motivation and access could not have been better, and it has helped my applicants before and since. Nevertheless, my advocacy for Liza hit a stone wall at that school. Frankly, if that one subscore were 6 points higher, and all else the same, that school would have been wooing Liza: she was such a strong applicant and so well-suited to their mission, as well as their ideal model of a medical student.

The takeaway from the cases of Emily and Liza is that the family network influences are not necessarily sourced in power, money or social hierarchy. They are far more likely and far more frequently rooted in community and professional networks, where people feel reciprocity and just want to help each other's kids reach their dreams.

Medical school admissions committee chairs, who are usually practicing physicians, often push away those we can think of as the "entitled influencers," people who are not asking for a closer review, but fully expecting that their request will get their applicant accepted at the school. Physician decision makers may push away a would-be influencer, even when they have to pay a professional price for it, as a matter of fundamental integrity and fairness in admissions. One admissions dean, who was near retirement at the time, told me that his committee rejected, without interview, the granddaughter of his most revered lifelong mentor. The mentor, who had served on the faculty of this school as a researcher, clinical faculty and administrator for his entire career, had reached out to my friend, the dean, several times, seeking the favor of an interview for his granddaughter. The granddaughter didn't come close to meeting the basic cutoff numbers, nor the requisite experiential background for the committee to consider her. My friend, whose experience had taught him to avoid what he called "courtesy interviews," recommended rejection. His mentor felt betrayed, initiated a bitter and angry discussion, and the decision effectively ended their relationship.

A decade earlier, that dean at that school rejected an applicant whom I thought deserved an interview. I had a strong feeling about it. When the cycle was over, I asked the dean to explain why the committee rejected my applicant. He reviewed the application and told me that it had clearly been a mistake. I remember so vividly him telling me that mistakes happen all too often. His school had way over 10,000 applicants for way under 200 spots. They had way under the number of admissions file reviewers he wished he had. He offered this as a form of apology and a request for understanding. He offered me that if the applicant did not have any success in that cycle that he would like him to reapply, and the dean would make sure he was reviewed wholly and completely. In fact, my applicant was not accepted anywhere, did reapply, and was interviewed and subsequently accepted at that same school by that same dean's admissions committee.

You might wonder why my applicant was not accepted anywhere if he was all that great. He was married with children and only applied to the four medical schools proximate to where his wife worked and extended family lived. He was the best fit by far for the school where I advocated for him, because he was a non-traditional applicant, completely primary-care and healthcare-equity focused, not research-oriented, and medicine would be a second career. He had a weak academic start in college, graduated and worked in healthcare for several years, and completed a two-year, highly respected postbac program with a 4.0. He had a strong MCAT, great experience, and stellar letters from faculty who had taught him, his community service mentors, and his clinical work employers.

Let's revisit the ideas of access, motivation and logistical strategy to give you a sense of how to apply them in a system with rules that can often seem random and arbitrary.

Access, Motivation and Timing

As I said above, one way to frame this working of connections is to think of two key aspects that an advocate can present—access and motivation—and then you can plan optimal timing.

Access is how close your contact is to the committee and what is the real nature of the contact's potential influence with the committee. Motivation is how much your contact wants to help you.

Why network or build professional connections? To increase your contact's motivation to help you and improve your access to the opportunities you want. Networking gives other people a chance to care about your premed and his goals. People associated with the world of medicine want to see others succeed in a medical field, so they in turn can help even more people.

When your connections care about your premed's dreams and commitment to a career in medicine, it motivates your them to find ways to increase your premed's access to resources, information, or medical school admissions staff. Motivation is a function of how much the contact really deep down wants to help your premed get into medical school and how much of their own social capital or other resources (time, perseverance) they are willing to devote to the project. Access is your contact's ability to influence medical school admissions by asking the committee to take a closer look at your premed's application, either in person or through a letter.

If you want to start the campaign before the admissions cycle begins, it is your aim to warm up those connections, not to push for your premed overtly. If the connections ask or make an offer to help, that gesture signals that they are motivated, which is good. At that point, you can subtly evaluate them. It's kind of awkward to be evaluating someone who has offered to help you. You want to enact this with the utmost kindness and discretion, but doing it is non-negotiable. You can start by asking for their advice on how to strategically approach decision makers. This gives you a better sense of them, their level of influence, and their understanding of how things work in admissions. The last thing you want to do is hurt your premed, or introduce more anxiety into their life because your effort to help was not helpful. You don't want your outreach to require them to clean up an issue that you initiated.

Weeding Out Uncle Wally

Families naturally find it interesting to talk about how their premed is faring in the process and the person they are talking to may feel like they would like to help. Perhaps it's a relative or a co-worker who has had a longstanding warm relationship with your premed. Many people like to feel that they can have an impact through back-door channels. It makes them feel good about themselves. Some people offer to advocate because they want to see if they have that kind of influence. How they have built and sustained their connections will determine their ability to help your premed.

It's really important not to accept all comers and give them carte blanche to reach out in any way that they like. This is not a "the more, the better" situation. In a sense, the person who wants to help needs to listen to you, and to do it the way and in the time frame that you suggest for it to make a difference. Your premed needs to supply something on paper with talking points the advocate can get his mouth around. They need, for example, to describe their relationship in a way that sounds professional, not strictly personal. *Winging it is not welcome, Uncle Wally.* If the contact doesn't want to comply, it might portend that they could actually dampen your premed's chances. You need to be careful about this, remembering whose life this is influencing—or messing with.

Connections That Don't Work

Failure to realize that not all outreach is useful or helpful, and can be, in fact, harmful, is one reason why parents and family members are subjected to distancing and obfuscation by institutions and even their own premed applicants. Don't be one of those people who barges in and makes their advocacy self-centered and self-serving. And do not do someone the favor of saying they can help your premed because you want to warm up your own relationship with them or because you feel awkward declining their assistance. Your premed will have trouble forgiving you for that because you will have made it harder to get into medical school—and it's hard enough already.

Maybe you need an introduction to others who have more or better access to committee members. Remember that it's a committee and thus fraught with political considerations. If an overly assertive or aggressive action takes place, or if the approach does not include knowledge of the admissions cycle or the applicant's strengths, it's bad for the applicant. The way that the contact intervenes can make or break the outcome. It can help the applicant get over a "hung" vote on the committee or it can doom her application.

Watch out for contacts known to many. You want to avoid depending on a contact who finds oneself in an awkward position because more than 2-3 people ask for advocacy at the same school, or a contact who just wants to see how much influence they have by testing the waters without really having a sense of the applicant's distinctive qualities.

Some people with influence just like to offer to throw it around to show off, and that could work or it could backfire. No toiling-away admissions person likes to get a call from a faculty member or administrator asking for special privileges. You do not want the influencer to advocate as a "favor" to you or to them, because then the applicant gets associated with special privilege over others, and that can really annoy some others on the committee who want to make a case for eradicating the hidden effects of privilege in their admissions process. Others resist the "favor" gesture just to assert their own moral superiority. That's a real doomer-move.

While unfair advantage exists in all admissions processes, remember that the unfairness is in the eye of the beholder. You cannot change, control, manipulate, correct through litigation, or even trust yourself to rationally understand and see unfairness in medical school admissions. Medical school admissions is singular among admissions programs because doctors have life and death responsibilities. Admissions officers see themselves as sacred gatekeepers in this regard, and they really detest political intervention.

It can backfire to get recommendations from people who hold worldly importance—the senator, president, famous person—any sniff of hoping for unfair advantage from a power perspective can send your premed's application into the compost pile. Instead, coach your premed to do the work of building significant relationships with people who are entrusted to guide, educate and lead them to develop into the physicians they hope to become. These people will rise to become knowing, caring and staunch advocates for your premeds and the best help you can find to secure the most favorable admissions chances. There is really no shortcut to medical school admissions success through the world of power and fame.

Setting Up Successful Advocacy

You, as the person seeking the help of the contact, can respond to their offer of help by asking: *What do you think is the best way to do this? Do you call or write a letter? Would you like to meet the applicant?*

The latter is best for starters, because once they spend a little time with the applicant, they will be motivated with greater integrity. They won't just be doing a colleague a favor, they will be advocating for the person they met, the applicant. In my experience, admissions officers want the person seeking special influence to really know the applicant and to be able to speak to their fine qualities from direct experience. The advocate needs to be prepared with talking points about your applicant and her suitability for that school.

The advocate should only contact the admissions office after your premed's application is complete with the school. Admissions officers do not have the bandwidth to flag an incomplete or non-existent file or start a tickler file to wait for an applicant's full record to show up. They need to be able to turn to a completed file that is ready for prescreen or committee review (AMCAS/AACOMAS/OMSAS/TMDSAS submitted and verified, secondaries submitted, letters received, all testing done, including Altus Assessments and the AAMC SJT, if they require it) and only then will they affix that all-important asterisk if they want to.

Networking With a High Access Contact

A high access contact is someone who has a warm and direct contact with a decision maker on the admissions committee. Your premed's first networking goal is to provide the contact with a sense of her as a person of substance and good character who is ready for medical school. Thus, it's good for them to meet and for your premed to be prepared for how to show up and talk about her plans at the meeting. She also needs to prepare for who she is meeting and show interest in their work and life.

Here is a short, scripted exercise you and your premed can use to practice breaking the ice at a networking meeting:

Hi, I am _____, great to meet you.

I am reaching out because my ___ mentioned that you are connected to ____ and I am applying to the ___ medical school.

How are you? How do you know them? How fascinating!

I wondered if you would help me by making an introduction?

Goodbye and thank you!

When introducing yourself to a new contact, whether in person or by email, explain why you chose to contact that person, what you know about them, and the distinctive value they have as part of your network. Highlight anything you share in common to start forming a bond, and then make a short, specific request of them. Finally, express polite and sincere gratitude for their time and consideration. Check to make sure your premed communicates in this way as well.

Networking As a Way of Life

The best networking plan is like a relay race. You start the race at an easy pace and you pass the baton for the home stretch. In your premed's high school years, it is not too early to begin to build your network. This gives your applicant great extracurricular and summer opportunities, which help them to choose a good college and helps the good college choose them. It allows them to see if medicine is a fit before they subject their liberal arts years to the demands of the medical school prerequisites. It gives you a sense of satisfaction that you can still help your premed in non-material ways.

As you look for medical opportunities in your community affiliations, professional networks, historical circles (high school and college, for example), and pursue your own interests and initiatives, keep looking for people who know doctors socially and professionally themselves. Let your premed know that you are doing this as part of responsible parenting or elder oversight. Incidentally, as you share your network growth with them, they, as always happens, will use your role modeling as an incentive to grow their own networks. Your modeling is the most effective way to use networks to increase their chances of getting into medical school. In a later chapter, we will explain how your premed can and should build a network, identify all the touchstones for effective social professional networks, digital and otherwise, and name the inflection points when they should be prepared to deploy their network to leverage their candidacy for medical school.

One final note: I am well aware that this book, and particularly this chapter, may be read by my advising colleagues and admissions officers. My professional colleagues may wonder or even consider it unprofessional—or even out of integrity—to guide premed parents to use their social capital as a sort of side door to medical school. I regret that my position on this may be seen that way, but after years of observing this process, I think it's time for the nanny placement office managers and housekeepers of the world to know how to use their own connections to help their kids get where they want to go. The admissions process is more than competitive; the gatekeepers are too few and the applications too many for it to be a truly rational, or even a fair process. Parents need to provide more than financial backing; they can also give the gift of their friendships and professional associations.

6 What It Takes to Go to Medical School: The Ideal Scenario

In preparing this volume, I spent eight days one February hunkered down at a rural retreat center, scouring the "literature" of premed advising books. In one from the 1970s, an admissions director, Marvin Fogel, MD, quoted his colleague, a now long retired Associate Dean of Admissions from Weill Cornell Medicine, John Ribble, MD. Dr. Fogel asked, "What are you looking for in a prospective medical student?" Dr. Ribble replied:

> *To avoid the question is unacceptable, but to answer it adequately is nearly impossible... We seek something more than academic capability. We look for individual qualities of devotion to excellence, leadership, altruism, breadth of interests–all characteristics that have a nice sound and are hard to define.*[5]

In the years since, medical school admissions committees have worked with the American Association of Medical Colleges (the AAMC) to answer that question adequately as well as to

---

5 The Medical School Admission Adviser by Drs. Marvin Fogel and Mort Walker (1976 - out of print), Hawthorn Books, p. 33

operationally define the individual qualities Dr. Ribble cited, and many more. They call the resulting canon "The Core Competencies for Entering Medical Students." Increasingly, these are used in holistic screening, in composing and evaluating the secondary essays, and in generating interview questions. Applicants need to study these competencies and reflect in depth on how each one applies to their own record. They will need to relate vignettes and stories that pithily provide evidence for their development of the competencies. The best way to do this is to spend time before applications open reflecting on their narrative—the stories and themes that combine to express who they are to the admissions office.

"Build medical school narrative" is not visible on most premed checklists, because no medical schools officially recommend or require it. But if you need further convincing that the applicant is required—not just recommended—to understand and use the competencies to highlight their medical school narrative, kindly read the contemporary words of Admissions Dean David D. Grier, MD, Associate Dean for Student Admissions, Wake Forest School of Medicine, from the AAMC website for applicants:

> *At the core of any patient encounter, there is a story. As physicians, we are primed to listen to stories, so a good story is key when a physician reads a medical school application or evaluates answers during the interview. Most medical school applicants have enough volunteer, work, shadowing, and research experiences to fill every space in their AMCAS application and prompt in their secondary applications. However, while many are very good at accumulating experiences, they are sometimes not so good at putting these experiences in context or effectively communicating them to interviewers and application reviewers. The applicant should be able to put all his or her experiences into the context of why they want to be a physician and describe their journey. Novelists, English professors, and screenwriters call this the 'arc of the story.' For example, the arc could be that a topic in class led to a research opportunity that led to a showing experience that*

then led to working with a group that is involved in that issue. This is different from the applicant that has a dozen unrelated experiences and is unable to connect them. In short, the applicant should be able to tell a good story that makes sense and engages the interviewer or reviewer rather than give a checklist of research, shadowing, and volunteering. Most applicants will not have a perfect story where everything falls into place, but that is OK. The most interesting stories have lots of twists and turns.

~David D. Grier, MD, Associate Dean for Student Admissions, Wake Forest School of Medicine[6]

The Ideal Scenario

An ideal applicant needs to be well-rounded, well-grounded and well-surrounded. ~Chere Pereira, retired premed advisor, Oregon State University

The ubiquitous "premed checklist" provides the essential minimum elements for readiness to apply to medical school. While I know plenty of premeds who got into a medical school without having one or even a few of those essential minimum requirements, I want to start here by covering the ideal, the best-case scenario, the perspective that you can adopt to guide your premed through the culmination of all his hard work and self-sacrifice. Your premed deserves some choice among schools at the end of the application cycle. To ensure this requires a robust set of credentials documenting the path of an emotionally and psychosocially well-developed human being with regard, one who is mature and at ease with adult living. This takes time.

Timing of the Application

While families often resist the idea of graduating college and not attending school while applying, this has become a common

---

[6] From AAMC Article: What Admission Officers Wish Premeds Knew Before Applying

trend. So many time consuming, resource-heavy milestones need to be in the evidence bag at the time of application, it takes a miraculously optimal set of circumstances for them all to be done by the end of junior year of college. A few of these milestones include an MCAT score, significant progress in substantive extracurricular activities that document service, teamwork, grit, an informed perspective on physicianship, and a strong academic record.

The optimal time to apply is not at the end of the junior year, or even the senior year for that matter. The optimal time to begin to prepare the application is after graduation from college. It's wiser to start with the plan of submitting the application a year after graduation. Don't start too early and encourage them to "just give it a try." To miss a deadline and extend the process is more discouraging than starting with an eminently achievable plan and then adjusting it if you complete items ahead of time. Remember when planning, that confidence is of inestimable importance.

When premeds apply in the summer after junior year, the MCAT timing has supplied them with plenty of stress on top of everything else they are juggling. It has taken a huge bite out of their opportunities to delve into the world of medicine, service and scholarly inquiry. Instead of exploring their medicine-related initiatives, they have prepared for a momentous and difficult test during their "spare" time. As the first semester of the senior year gets underway, the fortunate ones who really were quite ready and did everything according to plan, are getting invited to interviews. Of course that is an exciting outcome of years of hard work. Unfortunately, they then have to shift out of all those great habits and zeal for learning as they are offered midweek interviews, either online or in far-away destinations, which compels them to prepare for the interview, miss classes, reschedule exams and project deadlines, sacrifice scholarly activities and weekend events they only have one last opportunity in college to attend. At the same time, they need to come up with thousands of dollars to fund their jaunts.[7]

The less fortunate college seniors have to endure watching their classmates go off on interviews to which they have not yet been invited. Everybody is intensely curious about everybody else's outcomes and they check their phones ten, twenty, forty times a day for any meager sliver of information. I am not exaggerating. Some people compartmentalize friendships, never sharing the progress towards medical school with each other, because it's too painful. Some say in retrospect that applying while in college was a truly horrible way to waste the fall term of their last year in college, whether they were running to interviews every week or not, even whether they were accepted at a medical school or not: both ways, it "kinda' stinks."

When the premed applies during the senior, rather than the junior year, the MCAT stress hangover issue may apply. In addition, they sacrifice their last semester of college to the slavish process of preparing their primary applications. Just when they are completing capstone activities, like a research thesis, a huge club event, turning over leadership to a younger mentee, saying goodbye to friends they have studied with, loved and laughed with for four years, preparing their final exams to secure their final GPA, they are smothered by the demands of the primary application process, which must be ready in late May and sandwiched in between final papers and major exams.

For juniors, the premed admissions process severely compromises at least the fall semester of their senior year. For seniors, it compromises at least the spring semester. College is such a precious period of one's life and nobody deserves to have

---

7 When the coronavirus necessitated virtual interviews, it saved both applicants and schools a lot of money. This was good in the short term for those interviewing while in college or working full time jobs. Yet it degraded the interviewing/recruiting process and in-person optional interviews began to appear in the 2022 cycle.

a great, happy, celebratory and educationally rich senior year more than our dedicated, young physicians-to-be. And nobody is better poised to get a great one or two year job in teaching or research than a premed graduate. Who would not want to make productive use of all that intelligence, know-how and internal drive more than a busy clinic coordinator, medical research lab professor, teaching hospital or inner city school administrator?

No wonder advisors watch this at close hand and want to say to you, their families: *Let us all give these people a break!* In addition, in my many years of watching this process, I have yet to hear of one ounce of regret from a premed who took a gap year or two. Instead, they express jubilation and it does not tamp down their determination one iota. Medical schools appreciate premeds who have adapted to adult life and come to medical school as adults; they get the admissions edge. As Jane Cary, former advisor at Princeton University and Williams College, among others, once put it: *The gap year applicants muscle out the undergrad applicants on interview day.* In addition, parents often appreciate the economic reprieve of having a dependent working for a living between college and medical school, as well as the opportunity to enjoy their offspring for an extended period when they are not "too busy" to show up for their family.

Finally, it's just better in many ways to make a good decision far enough in advance that life settles down and people can plan. Parents can help plan this next major expense in their offspring's life. An applicant holding down a real job for two years can contribute financially. The cost of a medical school application cycle soars easily into the many thousands of dollars range.

Thus, while I have seen many who applied in the spring of junior or senior year do just fine, I vote for, at least initially, **planning on** a two-year gap for the reasons above, which means that your premed would submit their application to medical school in May, one year after graduating. I discuss ideas for gap year activities in a later chapter.

Metrics

While the higher the better, the realistic view on metrics is this. Ideally, a candidate has more As (~75% As) than Bs (~25%) in all science courses. The other grades average above 3.6. Only As and Bs appear on the transcript, no Ps, not Ss, not Ws, not INCs, and certainly not Ds, Us or Fs.[8] What about Cs? An isolated grade C+ or C in the first two years of undergraduate study, while certainly not ideal, is usually going to pass muster. A C- is often considered a failing grade because pass-fail courses often start the F at that threshold.

The applicant has taken upper level biology courses and done well. There should be semesters where they did well with many difficult science courses together. The choice of major does not matter. The student's interest in completing multiple majors and minors is not of interest to medical schools. Their eclectic interests and how they have pursued them are of far greater appeal and interest. These are shown in the narrative and by how they chose to spend their time outside of the classroom. Even perfect grades cannot make up for pursuing a thin trail or worse, no extracurriculars during college.

Individual schools, for a host of reasons, view the MCAT score differently. In general, if you get 127 minimum on each section, and a total score of 512, you are in range for staying in the screening system long enough to get noticed, provided your non-academic factors are substantive.

Service is Essential

The ideal applicant pursues innately driven initiatives that include service to others. Note that the word "passion" is often deployed in essays long after the original impulse that informed it has

---

8 Because some colleges mandated pass-fail grading during the pandemic, those grades during that time period are generally accepted by medical school admissions offices.

fizzled out due to the pressures of time and energy management during the long trek toward medical school. I think of passion as energy. When something you do gives you more energy than it drains you, on balance, it's a passion. Passions include music and athletics. It includes engaging in work that sometimes, even if unreliably, produces that ineffable feeling of being rewarded by the accomplishments of other people. Sophie was a star student at Cornell, who expected nothing less than an A in every course, no matter how challenging and competitive, and she managed it with hard, strategic, often joyless but consistent work. When her incarcerated mentee, Amber, passed basic math principles at the local GED program on the second try, Sophie's joy and pride in Amber's accomplishment was uncontainable. As was mine when that first medical school called Sophie to accept her into its first year class.

To engage in service is to actually work toward the benefit of others. To enjoy that service, it helps if the service fits into one's narrative and if the actual work a person does inspires, energizes and rewards them. Your inspiration is not everyone's. Your premed needs to find it and be willing to disengage from service activities that leave her feeling affect-flattened, drained and unrewarded. One rule of thumb is that the more proximate the applicant is to the same community or individual over time, the better she gets to know the human beings she is helping, the greater the chance that service will become a passion and be viewed as impressive by the medical schools.

On the other end of impressing medical schools, Greek Life has chapter officer titles designed to sound like the office holders are leaders who direct service initiatives, but most medical schools view a fraternity or sorority experience title as light and perhaps more about fraternal camaraderie than actually serving people. The same is unfortunately true for premed clubs, even though they can take considerable leadership skill to run and keep relevant.

The ideal applicant has continuous service at some level for the three years before the planned matriculation date for medical school. When the service includes direct impact on marginalized people and communities, when it involves teamwork and problem solving, challenges and determination to resolve them, and increasing leadership of others to encourage their service at the level of greatest impact and efficiency, that service goes a long way toward impressing the medical schools. This kind of experience is more important in the qualifying process than research.

Research Counts

Of course research counts. Research reveals a lot about applicants. It shows curiosity, problem solving, independence, determination, reliability, collaborative spirit and the willingness to learn on your own. Keep in mind that an important reason that medical schools are interested in applicant research is not really about the work itself or the skills one gains. Research labs on campuses are microcosms of the larger learning unit that is a university. A person who joins a lab as a young undergraduate is part of a group, often composed of lab managers, post docs, graduate students and faculty members who relate to each other with far more constancy and familiarity than undergraduates enjoy in their courses.

The recommendation letter that documents the applicant's research experience is frequently far more knowledgeable and revealing than any other regarding the applicant's integrity, reliability, dependability, productivity, collaborative spirit, intellectual curiosity and affability. If your applicant attends a large school with hundreds of prehealth professions students, a research lab is the place to find an intellectual home with true mentors and role models. The ideal applicant has made and sustained strong connections with at least a few faculty members and the lab is the place to get it. Thus students should choose a lab that has a warm and inclusive culture with people who like to mentor undergraduates. This is actually more important than the topic of study.

The applicant does not have to do bench research in life sciences. They can do anything in any field that has a research group.

What's important are the skills they exhibit and develop, their willingness to be reliably and dependably of service to the larger enterprise, and the interpersonal connections they forge and maintain.

The Family Support System Matters

The ideal applicant has abundant personal support in place for the application cycle. Family support means being ready to witness the whole process without judgment. Judgment includes offering unsolicited advising. Most premeds are monitoring themselves inwardly most of the time. They are measuring themselves by the achievements of others, and most often, feeling they have come up short. They use up cognitive space in their lives imagining they are not enough and getting anxious and downhearted about it. The most important light I can shed on this conditioned mindset is just to notice that regardless of all this negative mental undertow, they never give up. The ideal applicant never gives up, despite self-doubts, obstacles, challenges and setbacks.

From the family perspective, this can be confusing and paradoxical: *If it's so hard, why not do something easier with all your gifts, skills, talent and brains? Why spend all this money and all this time chasing a career that is so competitive and grueling?* These questions may come up for you, but they are not the right ones to ask, even to yourself. The ideal applicant never gives up because they are deeply and intimately connected to a powerful calling to be in an environment where heart, mind and spirit are all hooked up to the enterprise of healing others, along with kindred spirits who share that calling. And if that sounds too idealistic for you, I am talking about the core values of all physicians. Even though we have a health care system that burns off compassion and undermines the work-life balance, one that exhausts people while they are training to become doctors and often throughout their careers, at the core, that's where your applicant is coming from and heading towards. To suggest any alternative, you are inviting them to see you as unsupportive of their dreams.

Competent Advising Helps

I won't forget the time I attended an AAMC conference workshop for medical students on applying for residencies. After it concluded, I attended a reception where I noticed a medical student who had asked a great question in the workshop. I struck up a conversation with him about his question and a lively discussion ensued.

He asked me what I did and when I responded, *I'm a premed advisor!* his face dropped and this fourth year medical student soberly replied, *Are you going to crap on me now?* Some premeds consider their health career advisors to be dream-crushers, a fact that is pretty crushing for the advisors themselves. This is because of times when the advisors, in their 20-minute appointments, try to be frank about the ways that applicant records may deviate downward from the ideal scenario of the applicant who is ready to apply in this cycle to medical school. It is also because most undergraduate prehealth advising offices are understaffed, and the role of premed advising is misunderstood by their supervisors and administrators. Thus advisors often act as gatekeepers rather than facilitators and do not have the time, and sometimes perhaps the expertise, to convey individualized, helpful information. I mention this briefly because as a parent or family member, you don't want ever to pass judgment on the dream or even the way the person is going about it. Try to take criticism of the prehealth advisor as symptomatic of a systemic issue, rather than something to fix.

In a later chapter, I will talk about all the ways that advisors are invaluable on the journey to medical school. As you read this book, you will gain a sense of how much a seasoned advisor needs to know to guide a premed to medical school.

I hope that this information will help you to become that seasoned advisor for your premed.

Being Well-Grounded

The ideal applicant is grounded in her narrative, passions, and goals. She understands the themes and vignettes that illuminated her path to medical school. She knows how to present herself on forms, in response to particular questions, in an open-ended way and in an elevator speech. She knows how to conduct her end of a conversation so her themes and narrative stand out in high relief. She may not know this in December before she applies in May, but she needs to have the time and resources to learn it. The ideal applicant knows and appreciates her narrative, understands its structural integrity and how her attributes and experiences highlight it. She has a stable and supportive social life, certainty about the financial resources she will need, and the inner confidence and emotional stamina it takes to get through a year and a half of being one quarter of a centimeter away from seizing that elusive seat in medical school that she will ride to the future she has dreamed of pursuing.

Affording the Application Process

The application process for medical school is costly. Every act on the path has a fee attached: Things that require money beyond college tuition include:

- MCAT and MCAT prep
- Primary and secondary applications
- Travel for interviews, if allowed
- Cost of any activity that will help your student's application

How can parents and premeds get help affording the process? The central application services, AMCAS (American Medical College Application Service) and AACOMAS (American Association of Colleges of Osteopathic Medicine Application Service), for example, offer fee assistance for families who fit their income guidelines. Usually, if an applicant qualifies for this, as described on their website, they can simply inform the schools where they apply and receive waivers of secondary application fees.

How do I understand what the costs of medical school are? It's useful to have a budget in hand for the admissions cycle. Roughly estimated, you can expect it to cost $5,000 for the basic fees. If you hire a premed advisor independently, your applicant has the opportunity to travel for interviews and visit the campus on days for accepted students, and your applicant is accepted to a medical school and needs to pay a deposit, it will cost at least $10,000, but likely more.

Aside from the outlay of funds, premeds often cannot earn money. They cannot spare time to work at paid employment during school or in the summer and still maintain progress toward fulfilling the academic and extracurricular demands of preparing for medical school. Those who do work and manage to complete all the requirements are considered strong candidates for medical school. It's unusual and shows their independence and character.

It takes planning, budgeting and a lot of work in many different areas to successfully earn a spot in medical school. Parents can help develop a plan that is detailed and comprehensive. Good planning can save time and money, and encourage wellness in your premed.

7 High School and the Transition to College

As a rule, medical schools are not very interested in high school experiences and activities. It may be worthwhile for your premed to mention major activities like their life on a kibbutz in Israel, working ski patrol in the mountains of Colorado, Intel awards and major motion pictures they starred in, but otherwise, all your premed did there was become a pastel background to the person they are today and are becoming in college or afterwards. The greatest topic of interest to medical schools before college years, honestly, is your family's socioeconomic status and ethnic makeup, as well as how your premed personally identifies in distinctive but categorical ways, such as their racial mixture, sexual orientation, gender identity, the overall quality of their education/schooling before college, as well as any life influences or events that inspired your premed to become passionate about pursuing a career in medicine.

Train the Networking Muscle in High School

Premeds can begin to learn networking in high school. Not every high school premed ends up in medical school—and that's a good thing. If they get to see some of the gritty decisions and suffering that the field includes, it will only temper their resolve, or send them into genuine reflection about other great paths through adulthood. Premeds undergo a self-sorting process and many challenges must be braved along the way. I do hope that everyone who really feels called to medicine has the chance to become a doctor. Making sure that happens is central to my life purpose.

I recommend that high school students be made aware of the networks around them, and how they can work to everyone's benefit. We all socialize, but when we see how our social networks facilitate our professional development, we can begin to pay more attention to them, nurturing them and recognizing how we all depend on each other to reach our potential. When your offspring feels dragged to a social event with you, stop the train and remind them that they might meet someone there who can facilitate or at least ease their medical school admissions path. Adolescents seek autonomy and need you to teach them to discern the difference between networking and unethical influence. If you use your social capital to open doors for them, they still need to learn how to keep that door open all by themselves.

Keep in mind, always, that the best networking is 100% genuine, where you are simply getting to know new people because you're genuinely curious about them, offering to help or are seeking information or advice, without intimating a desire for a specific outcome. No one likes to feel like you are meeting them just because you want to use them later. This is why it is also good to start early before you need to start asking for favors!

It's great if your premed can spend time after school outside of her comfort zone (but not outside of yours of course!). By this, I mean working with adults in a research lab where her contributions are needed and expected or by serving a population different from the one she grew up with on a sustained, frequent basis. I don't mean by this to signal that all premeds are well-off and should spend time with those who aren't. If the premed is not well off, she can get a job at the country club. Recently, as I write this, one of my applicants got a coveted interview invitation from an elderly man whom she served regularly for lunch at his country club. During her gap year, she holds a full time job and a weekend job to cover her application expenses. When he asked her about her aspirations and she told him her background, he asked his son to have a phone call with her. His son is a physician on a medical school admissions committee where she recently applied and dreamed of attending.

It's important to see in high school that we indeed live in a stratified society, and this becomes concrete and visible through our direct experience. It's edifying to immerse oneself in any unfamiliar culture. By assuming a helping role, your premed can develop the curiosity and awareness he will need to understand these problems more deeply than at the purely intellectual level explored in college. Later, he will be equipped to address inequality in access to healthcare as a doctor.

If he works in a scientific research lab as a high school student, he will learn experimental skills and earn commendations that will allow him to qualify for a research lab in college that will teach him even more, allow him to work independently on research, and provide a good letter of recommendation if he's deserving. It's so important to be selective about the lab he joins. The people there should be kind, open and mentoring. Labs that have a competitive, silo-ing, publication-factory vibe are to be avoided. It will be a negative experience, and particularly during the high school years, you don't need to choose a lab based on what it is researching. Choose it for the good people.

Advice About Choosing an Undergraduate School

In general, a small college is better academically for any student than a large school because at a small school, prerequisite courses will have fewer students and a lower student to teacher ratio.

At a smaller school, a student will learn to show what they know in ways beyond multiple choice tests, probably through a combination of essays and oral exams—they'll be able to show what they learn in different ways. When they get to the point where they are applying to jobs and medical schools, more narrative forms of showing what they know will serve them well in presenting themselves to others. Students often crave large schools because there are more students and more opportunities. But in terms of academics, it is pretty clear that small schools are better for students than large schools.

You might question if large, highly competitive, selective schools such as the University of Michigan, Stanford, or Cornell might be better for a student in terms of the medical school application than a small and lesser known school like a regional state school. A person who goes to a regional state school campus is able to shine to their faculty members much more easily than at larger schools. They are likely to have an easier time developing relationships with professors and receiving distinctive and compelling recommendation letters for their application. Medical schools want to recruit students who achieve high at their school, whether their school is small, little known, publicly funded, or large, famous, and selective. What matters is that the students are doing well and near the top of their class.

Finally, there are a couple of specific undergraduate medical programs that a premed should be aware of. Programs that offer a BS/MD or BS/DO degree give the premed a conditional guarantee of admission to medical school and college in one exciting acceptance letter, and a shortened period for finishing medical school. Some medical schools in other countries routinely accept students to medical school straight out of high school. In Mexico, for example, UAG School of Medicine in Guadalajara does this, and it even has a special program for Americans and Canadians that is a lot cheaper than our traditional routes to medical school. A premed can apply there, or to any number of other countries with similar training systems for their citizens, go through their medical school, take the US or Canadian licensing exams, and apply for residency in the US. I have seen this. I think it's sad to forego college to go to medical school, but such a path has its own life changing growth possibilities!

The "Goodbye Honey" Talk

You and your premed need a plan to make medical study a reality. Effective planners are more successful than others. It's that simple. The plan unfolds over many years in a very young life and like your GPS system, needs to have room for re-routing. So, what is the standard plan? Here's how you could describe it to your premed as you have your final talk before leaving her sitting on her twin XL dorm bed dressed with new sheets and decorated with the old pink comforter that is destined to become either ditched or crumpled in a permanent heap within weeks of your departure.

Here's what to say:

The Message: Build Relationships Now

In the first semester of college, take it easy on the academics and let yourself become accustomed to the undergraduate culture. Make colleagues. Premeds need colleagues, role models, mentors and unflagging family support. You can and will also make friends, but that's not the most important social "work" of the freshman year.

A colleague is someone who has similar aspirations and shares your sense of the qualities of character needed to get there—discipline, perseverance, professionalism, and personal integrity. These people will form your study groups, your lab partnerships, your research assistants, and your support system on the ground. Role models are more advanced students whom you will meet in student activities, campus events, advising offices, and elective classes. Be proactive in developing these relationships as these people can give you vital information on what courses to avoid and to take, what labs are good to work in, what course schedules are brutal or manageable, and they may even be available for the occasional midnight tutoring session.

Mentors are people who are further along the path than you are: your TAs, grad students in the lab, staff advisors, and most important, faculty. In the first semester, you need to find ways to make professional relationships with faculty members and staff advisors. For your entire career, these people will form a network of crucial assistance to you. The most obvious function of faculty is that they serve as the references that outsiders like employers, internship sponsors and medical schools see as ultimate authorities on your suitability for the opportunities you will seek throughout college and medical school. They will receive the emails and phone calls asking for an informal assessment of your professional and personal qualities. They will write the time-consuming labors of love also known as letters of recommendation. How well they seem to know you in those letters (and how much time they're willing to put in to make them great) can make or break your admissions chances to medical school. It takes time and shared experience to build these relationships, and your initiative, yours alone, will to a large degree, build these relationships. Do not neglect this as you become acculturated to college.

One more significant relationship of the freshman year is worth contemplating in advance, as part of the plan. Romance—of the fumbling beginner style is bound to happen, in your head, your body, the head and/or body of the object of your affections, and, if you are very fortunate, in your heart. Romance neither accelerates nor derails the premed path. It is a definite detour that I hope you enjoy. Write about it as you go through it, the pleasure and the pain. Your life is a reality show; reviewing your real-time recorded thoughts will help to inform your perspective on your undergraduate years when you have to share your reflections on those years, at the time of application to medical school. You are not going to write about your love life on your application, per se, but your love life and other welcome distractions will be in there, between the lines that explain the ups and downs of your academic performance and productivity."

The Message: The Boilerplate Academic Plan

Talk to your advisor about your academic plan. If your first advisor does not or cannot address your questions, find another advisor. If the college does not refer you, ask your professors. Ask your RA. Ask your classmates for the name of an advisor who helped them. Post your plea for relatable and expert advising on Facebook. Be persistent in getting the advising that fits you. You deserve it.

Here is what you need to discuss with the advisor: In the first five semesters, or eight quarters of college, you will attempt to plan a way to take all the premed prerequisites. These include generally retaking any AP Biology you took in high school.[9] *In addition, you will need statistics, biochemistry, chemistry (a minimum of three courses), a year of physics, and varying courses in the humanities, including composition, literature, and social science. You will need to balance your college and major requirements with medical school requirements. This can become complicated, because colleges don't plan curriculum to appease medical schools.*

Some take the medical school requirements into consideration.[10] *Others like to think they are preparing their science undergraduates for research careers. In addition, during the sixth semester or the ninth quarter, the end of the junior year, you can take a term away from campus in a foreign country or a domestic program that allows you to study and learn in a whole new way that will refresh your learning batteries and remind you of why you wanted to attend college and go to medical school in the first place. A sound academic plan will give you this freedom and once-in-a-lifetime opportunity. You can be a premed and enjoy college. Planning helps.*

Thus endeth The Talk, and now you really have to go home with your box of tissues. The "Goodbye, Honey" talk will let your premed see you as an authority in this process, someone willing to be consulted and to coach from the sidelines.

Communicating with Your College Student

I was once shown statistics at a student affairs division meeting at Cornell about the frequency with which students talk with their parents while away at college. The data were amusing in their predictability. Women talk with their moms the most, their dads

---

9 Sorry about that, everybody. Studies show that students who forgo the AP credits and take the college biology course get better grades in biochemistry and other advanced biology courses, and do better on the MCAT Biology section. This is because the AP curriculum is not designed to transition seamlessly to upper level coursework. That's the job of the college curriculum planners.

10 This curricular consideration is actually a useful selection criteria for choosing an undergraduate school.

second most, followed by male students who talk to their mom, and finally, sons talk with their dads the least. Some families plan to set aside time when all can be free, such as a late afternoon on a weekend day for a video meeting. Sometimes the family will play a game or do a crossword, sometimes just catch up and talk. To set a plan like this allows you to hold your worries and concerns, your ideas and your curiosity until the agreed upon time. It allows your premed to tuck things away for that time.

In my generation, college students were expected to write home once a week. Sometimes it was a drag, and sometimes the content glossed over what really mattered to me, but that weekly check-in ritual, with its ruminative and reflective aspects, was really useful for learning how to talk about, and reflect on, my experiences and feelings. The video call is an apt modern substitute for this. In it, you should model talking about what matters, showing that you consider your offspring to be an independent adult, and you should also model open and honest listening. Let them talk on while you stay present to what lies beneath the surface. Only offer advice after seeking their permission and ask for their advice on your own dilemmas to reinforce how much you respect their views. There will be canceled weeks, boring weeks, freaky weeks and worried weeks. Interspersed with all this will be loving weeks where you see growth and independence that will make your heart sing. Establishing and insisting on these conversations will give your family strength and make your premed feel safe, soothed, seen and secure.[11]

---

11 Daniel J. Siegel, MD and Tina Payne Bryson, PhD (Do you really see your child? LinkedIn 2020)

8 How to Get Effective Prehealth Advising

Nearly all colleges and all special programs for medical school-bound college graduates have advisors. The main job of an advisor is to inform students of how they can navigate the college curriculum and internal opportunities to become well-educated. Over the decades, the college advisor job evolved from explaining how to get through a liberal arts curriculum to how to prepare for a professional career. Colleges vary a lot in their ability to help their students launch themselves into future careers. Sometimes, I wonder if they should be expected to do that, and if they give their advising staff adequate resources to fulfill that promise well.

The generic term for an advisor who specializes in any health career admissions process is "prehealth advisor." The institutional prehealth advisor's job is to know and understand what an applicant needs to do during their college years to be viable candidates for healthcare-related professions. The advisor needs to understand their college, its curriculum and coursework, and to know the faculty well enough to refer students to courses and to research opportunities in their labs. Advisors also need to know about and advertise special programs the college might offer to enhance the prehealth student's experiential background. Advisors need to know the community to guide premeds to get clinical engagement/observation and to do meaningful service. Often employers approach advisors to advertise their jobs.

Prehealth advising is a very different job at a small liberal arts college like Wells College or Barnard than it is at megaliths like Berkeley and Cornell. I know; I have worked for all four schools. In fact, have guided applicants from nearly 100 undergraduate schools. The smaller the school, the more likely the advisor is expected to master pre-law and pre-business, as well as prehealth. It is also more likely that the advisor is a science professor who gains a lighter teaching load for pitching in as their student body's prehealth advisor.

The bigger the school, the more transactional the advising becomes. Advisors are specialists in particular professional fields, but they often have 2500 advisees at all levels of college to work with. Transactional advising is brief. There's little nurturing or exploratory conversation. Advisors hold briefings attended by hundreds of students or teach a credit-bearing course on how to prepare for an application cycle to medical school. Students show up for their 15-minute appointments (that they waited six weeks to have) with their list of questions…it's a lot like going to the doctor these days!

The advisor may be a faculty member, a non-faculty academic advisor, or a dedicated prehealth advisor. Each type of advisor has strengths and weaknesses based on the role she assumes in the institution. For example, a biology professor who gets reduced teaching time to advise prehealth students may be stretched among her research, her teaching, and staying abreast of developments in the rapidly evolving field of prehealth admissions. She sees the same students in her courses as in her advising office. If the student doesn't relate well to her, it can be intimidating for the student to take advantage of that resource.

The same can be true of an academic advisor, whose central responsibility is to guide his students through the course curriculum, research-for-credit experiences, and service learning the institution provides its students. A dedicated prehealth advisor usually stays up with the field, but do they have time to really develop each applicant for four years? Do they really have the resources to care for and guide each person? Because one advisor who really stays in touch during the process can't really have more than 50 advisees, large undergraduate schools would need to hire dozens of full time prehealth advisors alone. Usually, prehealth advisors who advise specifically for health career applications only exist at schools with very high applicant volumes of 100-700 applicants annually.

Full disclosure: I am an independent premed advisor in private practice. Whereas once I earned a paycheck from a university to advise applicants applying to health career schools, now I earn my living directly from applicants whose families (with some exceptions) pay me. I also offer pro bono advising. While I acknowledge that I derived a great deal of pride in my outward facing role as a representative of a well-respected university that churned out over 400 applicants to medical school each year, the more I learned and the better I got at advising, the more that role did not allow me to serve our applicants nearly to the level of my intention, ability and knowhow. Over the years that I served the premeds, prevets, predents and pre-every-other-imaginable-health-career, I came to see that our applicants were actually underperforming in admissions, and that I was part of, and contributed to the assumption held naturally by parents that their children were actually receiving the best advising because they went to a prestigious university. That rationale simply was not supported by the institution's budget priorities. I still love that university and its students, many of whom now hire me privately to help them. I know now that most, if not all, universities really struggle to provide adequate, informed and accessible advising in every area from academic advising to career advising. It's a huge challenge, a complex and thorny problem and no one is to blame in the end.

Premed advisors like working with their students, but the realities of the institutional constraints they face prevent them from giving their premeds the time and focused attention that the medical school path demands. Often, they are asked abruptly to take on time-consuming jobs that arise temporarily, like serving on hiring committees. Or they have seasonal responsibilities like managing college recruiting fairs with endless organizational details to orchestrate. The sad disconnect between institutional luster and truly effective advising is widespread.

It is true at many, if not most, undergraduate schools: the larger the school, the more likely its premeds are not sufficiently advised to the degree that would allow them to benefit most from the education they are receiving. Advisors do their best, but the ratio of advisor to advisee is insurmountable. The schools are under-resourced in their advising. This is why I don't care to point the finger at the schools where I served: the problem is rampant.

Small liberal arts schools are challenged, as well, to provide good advising. The smaller the school, the more likely that the person doing the part-time advising is a faculty member who is juggling a heavy teaching load and does not have the time to learn anything of substance about the medical school admissions process. The reason it's sad is because parents footing the tuition bills and premeds footing the heavy curricular demands, just don't know how much better served they could be. They don't know at the outset of the admissions cycle that they won't fare as well because they may not know if they are learning what they need to know from their advisors. The independent advising arrangement works better for me at this stage of my career because there is no ambiguity about whose interests I am serving, which is my applicants, 100%.

Understanding Institutional Advising

Institutional advisors are pivot wheels between the institutional culture and the medical school culture. I loved that my university enrolled a truly stunningly diverse class, but that great initiative compounded the challenges I faced in tailoring my advising information to each person's situation. We had premed applicants who grew up as children of migrant field workers in Southern California, asylees from the Middle East, and children of Tibetan refugees who had grown up with parents who practiced Tibetan medicine. We enrolled students who were born in this country to illegal immigrants, and we had students whose parents lived 6000 miles away, were CEOs of multinational corporations, and had sent their children at age 13 to US boarding schools, never to live together as a family again. We had the children of Iowa farmers, Wall Street hedge fund owners, and someone whose dad sharpened 6-foot diameter blades at a Saskatchewan lumber mill for a living. We had students whose parents purchased houses for them to live in near campus when they were sophomores. We had students who drove Hummers and students who slept in other students' cars because they could not afford housing. We had students who lived from couch to couch, searching daily for events where free food was served because they couldn't afford a stash of ramen soup. Many do not realize how many US college students today are legitimately food insecure.

All these students wanted to become doctors and their educational savvy, opportunities for clinical engagement and service, and understanding of medical school admissions landed on as broad a spectrum as their backgrounds did. They needed time to talk over their emerging narratives, to discern their talents, strengths, weaknesses and areas to improve before applying. In my attempts to do this work with them, they taught me much more than I could ever hope to teach them. Yet I needed more time to work with them all effectively.

Add to this the destructive alcohol culture that sucks freshmen in like a Roomba on steroids, the underground trade in Adderall and other stimulants, the 800-person organic chemistry lectures that grade on the mean based on three multiple choice exams, and you have a sense of what advisors face in a diverse undergraduate climate. When all you have time to provide applicants are 45-minute *en masse* briefings on select advising topics and one or two 15-minute individual advising appointments each semester, the advisor needs more than professional development workshops on time and task management to meet the demand.

How can an advisor in this institutional setting possibly guide applicants to build their own unique narrative, convene a faculty committee to interview them for the purpose of preparing a truly insightful institutional letter (which medical schools ask for from undergraduate schools, but only about half can afford to provide)? How can they develop a meaningful list of schools, draft and redraft the personal statement, ditto for their secondary essays, prepare them for interviews, and guide them through the critical process of networking throughout the cycle so they can get interviews, get off waitlists and reach their maximal success?

The answer is that advisors can't do that, and most that I know would love to be able to. They would love to work on collaborative teams with other full time prehealth advisors, but many work alone, feeling that nobody else knows what they are doing at their institution. My point is this: It's damaging to a health career aspirant for an institution to go along with the parent and students' assumption that *one can* when **one can't**— or when the resources they need are simply not available. I am also explaining why you should not turn your disappointment toward the premed advisor. They are doing the best they can, and your premed should just sit down with them at the outset to clarify what they can and cannot do to help the premed get into medical school, take the good they offer, and find the other help the premed wants and/or needs outside of the institution. I want this book to help you know the truth, or at least, the critical factors, before you head to the internet.

Evaluating the Premed Advising at Your Student's College

How many applicants to medical school does this advisor work with? The more applicants, the more statistically-based their advice is, from necessity. Your premed is an individual and medical school admissions is not all a numbers game. It is increasingly holistic.

Does the institution pressure its advising staff, subtly or overtly, to have a high acceptance yield to post graduate programs? See the next question!

What percentage of applicants from the school go on to medical school? What percentage are successful in the first try? The higher the percentage, the less you should base your premed's prognosis on the advisor's opinion. What?! Why? The higher the percentages above the national average, the more their students are being intelligently and caringly redirected—or downright discouraged—from pursuing the intensely competitive medical school admissions route. This is just one of the many counter-intuitive elements you will encounter as you vicariously observe the premed admissions process. You may think that a high acceptance rate is a selection criterion for undergraduate admissions. Now I, as your advisor, am asking you, the premed parent: *Is that really true?* I suggest that you check that belief at the door.

Does the advisor need to know about every health career out there? If so, they may have only limited knowledge about medical school.

What proportion of health career applicants are applying for allopathic and osteopathic degrees? Is the advisor knowledgeable about allopathic and osteopathic medical school admissions? Do they have an outmoded (and thoroughly disproven stigma) about osteopathic medical schools?

Effective Communication with the Institutional Advisor

Advisors and admissions officers see themselves as the rational protectors of the admissions environment. They see parents as the irrational protectors of their children. You can never talk anyone into anything if they frame you as irrational and overly subjective regarding your cause, because they will invoke what they see as their morally superior, rational behavior—not because it actually **is** superior or rational, but because it is ultimately self-protective, **the** ultimate self-defense tool of the institution.

What the modern American research university really fundamentally wants, stands for, and how its mission statement should accurately read is: "Our mission in the 21st century is to legally protect ourselves from anyone and everyone who could possibly threaten us." We could debate how true this is, and if it is mostly true, how sad it is, but instead, let's be practical. The Family Education Rights Privacy Act, known as FERPA, plays a big role in how the institutional advisor interacts with parents and premeds. Advisors are often trained, in not required to invoke FERPA in refusing to speak with parents and other family members about their advisees. It's frustrating for you.

A few parents can permanently burn out an advisor from collaborating with parents, or even accepting their phone calls. One of my favorite examples came from an Oklahoma advisor, who told me about a freshman premed who brought their mother to a meeting during orientation. The mother wanted the meeting so she could give notice to the advisor that she did not want her son exposed to the theory of evolution in their science classes in college. My colleague, the advisor, leveled her piercing stare at the mother, and said softly: *Take a long look at this young man before you leave, because all kinds of evolution is about to take place inside of him at this university and there's not a thing you can do about it, Ma'am.*

Staff members at universities in all kinds of roles are essentially trained to stonewall parents when they call, or routinely refer them to a higher up, someone who usually has no familiarity with medical school admissions, but has read the communications manual, who knows exactly how the university counsel's office recommends that staff members communicate with families of their students. Given that FERPA is interpreted by most supervisors of prehealth advisors as "say nothing," and the university counsel's office cautions even supervisors against speaking with families, the spokespeople need a cover story that everyone can buy. They tell your premed that they are in college now and they should not need their parents to tell them what to do and how to do it. When parents call, they imply that their actions are meddlesome and intrusive. They use every fiber of independence-seeking in your premed to enlist their help in pushing you away and out of their affairs. This is great advice to many parents who may need to learn about boundaries in their own influence and neediness, but in my view, it's sad that universities sometimes use FERPA as a kind of a communication shield in this way. Medical school admissions is one of those processes in family development that most definitely takes a village—with open communication in all directions.

Every parent wants their offspring to become independent in college. Many parents are kind of done with, even bored with the hovercraft thing, and want to return to fully inhabiting their own lives and pursuing their own dreams when their kids go off to college. So it's all good. What I see as not good is when some advisors conclude that parents want to keep hovering, controlling, micromanaging every time they call. Sometimes the premed just needs a little help in understanding what was said and wants to lean on their parents for support again.

Here is a sturdy rule to impose on yourself: **Do NOT call the prehealth advisor**. When it comes to institutional advisors, at your premed's college, stay out of the direct conversation. Since you are likely not to be able to intervene directly, it's good to get in the habit of talking things over with your premed to guide them in how to learn the information they need from the premed advisor. Coach your premed to ask the advisors relevant and individualized questions—and help them to interpret any negative messages they think they hear. Don't let your premed waste the advisor's time asking questions that are on the website or available anywhere else.

Don't consult directly with the advisor yourself. Only call the school to advocate for your child or someone else's if you have good reason to fear that someone's life is in danger. If you have the slightest concern there may be a potential for a student to hurt himself or hurt others, you should absolutely contact the school without thinking twice.

Most college advisors are also back-breakingly over-occupied, and just cannot allot the time to welcome parent conversations.

In addition, parents sometimes spoil it for other parents when they call in moments of great emotional distress carrying false expectations about the responsibility or sphere of influence the advisor holds at the institution. When a parent calls the premed advisor to complain about a situation someone else has caused, it may make the advisor feel angry also, and powerless. Don't subject the advisor to that. Call an upper-level administrator. You may not get relief from your concern, but at least the upper level administrator has staff designated to "handle" you. They will take notes, and guess what: the notes become an education record that FERPA protects: your student has the right to request to see the notes later.

The Institutional Letter

Some advising offices compile the institutional letter, or committee letter, on behalf of applicants, which means that they interpret transcripts, resumes, questionnaires and letters of recommendation into a two-page narrative that highlights the applicant's virtues as they apply for a life in medicine. The committee or institutional letter is particular to medical (which includes podiatry, optometry and dental school) admissions. I have written these letters for three institutions for a total of fourteen long summers and know all their advantages and disadvantages more intimately than I would like, or even want to share.

Every school has its own unique system for compiling these letters and it's very good to know even when you are applying to college what system your prospective school uses. It's almost impossible to capture all the ways of producing a committee letter in a simple description, so I will "gravitate to the mean." Midway through the academic year, pre-applicants are required to essentially draft a rehearsal for the medical school application. This is one of the beneficial (albeit indirectly) outcomes of the committee letter process; it gets applicants started six months in advance. They answer questionnaires and list their activities and experiences, with date spans, locations, types of activity, and level of involvement, all noted in bullet and narrative form. Frequently these materials are sent to a faculty or staff volunteer (hence the term "committee") who interviews the pre-applicant and makes notes or drafts a letter, which is then polished and standardized by a member of the office staff or a hired editor.

There is a little hitch at this stage. Most advisors preview the student's transcripts and if the GPA is below a fixed level, they may set a previously unmentioned bar for the applicant to get past. They require an advising meeting before going forward, or they just write the applicant to tell them they don't qualify for a letter.

For that reason and to appear as inclusive and fair, most undergraduate schools claim that they write for everyone, but it's not really the case. Some of them write for everyone whom they have not been able to personally educate about their weak chances of admissions and whom they could not dissuade from applying. Others write for everyone who seeks a letter, but they write only brief and uninformative letters for people they think will have a hard time getting in. FERPA specifically prohibits universities from putting conditions on the receipt of an education record that the institution normally provides to any student matriculating for a degree (letters are education records, just like transcripts).

Why in the world do they do either of these things? They may tell themselves that they are doing the applicant a favor. Maybe they want to winnow the number of letters they write so they are not so inundated in the summer. Sometimes they may turn down a letter request at the expense of the applicant's confidence. They think they can estimate who will get in and who won't, so they don't want to waste their time and the applicant's money. Sometimes they intimate to an applicant that they will write negative letters for people who don't take their advice to withdraw the request for the committee letter, and sometimes they just write generic letters without informing the applicant. They do this in the name of objectivity. They don't have to worry about the consequences of damaging a person's chances to become a physician because they have intimidated every student into waiving their FERPA rights under what I consider somewhat false pretenses. These pretenses include warning them that medical schools do not trust applicants who want to retain their civil right, their FERPA right, to view their own letter, which is a bona fide education record.

The medical schools inform advisors that they want the committee letter to differentiate applicants, so they should compare them. The easiest way to compare the son of Tibetan immigrants to the daughter of an investment bank CEO is by GPA, or MCAT. Schools try to include all the interesting background stuff in the letter, but when it comes to the all-important final paragraph that compares their own students, head to head, as better or worse than each other, the medical schools urge them to rank their students. When they use GPA or MCAT in the committee letter ranking, I wonder if they really help the holistic review process. GPA is a number. How can it be used in such a difference-making way to define a person's suitability for a life in medicine?

For the applicant's perspective on the committee letter, I quote from **Into the Magic Shop**, a memoir by Stanford neurosurgeon, James R. Doty, where he recounts his experience with his university's committee[12]:

> *I dutifully went to see the premed committee secretary to schedule my interview. I can still see her clearly in my mind, as she pulled out my file, perused it briefly, then looked up at me in a dismissive fashion and ...said, "I'm not scheduling an interview for you. You'll never get into med school. It's just a waste of everyone's time." I stood there dumbfounded. Getting a letter from this committee was imperative. It was the first step....*
>
> *I took a deep breath. "I appreciate what you said, but I want an appointment."*

---

12 P. 163-164, Into the Magic Shop, February 2017

> *"I can't do that. You don't qualify."...*
>
> *"That's unacceptable."*
>
> *Eventually the secretary yielded, and Dr. Doty faced even more formidable opposition at the start of the interview.*
>
> *I walked in, looked around, and realized this wasn't a meeting. It was an inquisition. And I was the heretic.*
>
> *"...I believe this meeting is really a waste of time for everyone here. Can you convince us differently, Mr. Doty?... I appreciate that you forced the secretary to schedule this appointment, but expecting us to recommend you for a profession for which you have zero chance of success is the height of arrogance. Medical school is extremely competitive, which I'm sure you are aware, while your GPA is not."*
>
> *"I would like to say something," I said.... "Who gave you the right to destroy people's dreams?"*

Dr. Doty got his letter, the secretary (not the advisor or faculty) then directed him to a special program for low socioeconomic status (SES) applicants, he went there after college, and then was accepted to Tulane Medical School with his 2.5 UC Irvine GPA. Now that he is a neurosurgeon, he is not afraid to name names and to characterize his experience. I strongly recommend that you read his book. Unfortunately, most premeds will not speak up as he did, nor will they speak out later about how and why advisors and faculty committees may misuse their power over young lives as they did in his case, and why they have developed the mindset that they need to be gatekeepers to medical school. Advisors and undergraduate faculty are not the gatekeepers. Medical school admissions committees are the gatekeepers.

It's one thing for an advisor to tell an applicant that she can do more things and inevitably take more time to become a better applicant, a potentially more successful applicant. It's quite another to imply in any way that the applicant will not get into medical school this year or ever. It's so easy for a high-strung premed to feel that they just heard those terrible words from their advisor, even if the advisor didn't verbalize those exact words. And you will hear plenty of doctors telling you that's what they heard from their premed advisor. It's embarrassing, really, how often they hear that.

If your premed comes to you feeling discouraged by the premed advisor, always take this news first with full-out empathy, and unqualified emotional support: *That totally sucks, honey.* Let the feelings come out. Then ask questions to help them discern if they were actually told they can't be doctors ever, or if they were told there is good reason to wait to try. It's very hard for some premeds to tell the difference! Encourage them to go back to the premed advisor and give feedback: *When you said my GPA was too low, I heard you saying that I can't become a physician. Was that your intention?* If the advisor says yes, well, that's the end of that relationship. If the advisor says no, and wants to clarify, then you might want to encourage them to stick with the advisor.

Your premed needs to know that the job of the premed advisor is to help them. The premed advisor is not the admissions committee; their role is to support your premed's goals and dreams with information that they can use to get into medical school someday. It is not their job to give unsolicited tangential advice on other career paths. That's not your job either, incidentally. At the place where dreams are held and nurtured, inside of your premed, is where they truly are autonomous beings. It is up to them to be the first to look to alternatives, and it's nobody else's business.

But I digress. Committee letters are more and more frequently written by temporary workers, a fact undisclosed by the school, for obvious reasons. When advisors have the task of committee letter composing and disseminating in addition to everything else they do, even if they support the process to everyone around them, as the years go by, they will develop a secret revulsion for writing these letters. They might love writing one letter, but trust me; they hate writing the next one. Few people can write more than three in a whole work day. Letter writing takes up the best––and often extends into the worst—hours of your summer and they...never...end. Advisors talk amongst themselves and then often look for ways to convince their supervisors to fund temporary workers to write the letters. Obviously this means that your premed's letter is not written by someone who knows them well, which is key to a letter that really gets noticed. It may be later reviewed and edited by someone who knows the premed well, but composing a letter and reviewing it in a factory production line are not the same thing.

At schools that produce committee letters, the advisor's summers are filled to the brim with letter writing. They simply do not have time to advise applicants who are at the beginning of their all-important admissions cycle. Many schools hire English PhD students as temporary workers to review the primary application personal statement. The applicant gets one review. The personal statement is a truly evolutionary document. It takes many drafts, no matter how great it is to start. Premeds don't take many—if any—writing classes and should not be conditioned to think that two drafts will suffice for such an important document. In my view, the important advising on essay writing that the advisor is best positioned to do, and the all-important committee letter, are too often outsourced to people who may receive a few hours of training on how to do this job, and who barely understand the big picture. Further, applicants are usually instructed to avoid all communication with the advisor over the summer.

Clearly, the problem at our universities is insufficient staffing, but at the root of insufficient staffing are institutional priorities. Precious few institutions make it a priority to invest in best practice advising for medical school admissions, which is actually the most complex of all advising. They should admit it's a low priority. Part of the reason why this is so, is that few upper level administrators understand premed advising. They don't even seem to appreciate that physicians who were actually helped along their journey are more likely to give back to their undergraduate school when asked to donate and needing to choose between the undergraduate institution and the medical school they attended.

As a parent, you can't fix problems of this complexity and magnitude. Neither can your child's premed advisor. You do need to know that they exist, and you have a right to know exactly how institutional committee letters are produced, how much time the premed can hope to have one-on-one with their advisor leading up to and during the application cycle, and how the personal statement review is carried out by the school. This is an example of a situation where it may be a parent's role to intervene and ask the tough but fact-based questions about their premed's advising office. FERPA cannot be used as a shield because you are not seeking confidential education record information about your applicant.

Think of it: How awkward and self-destructive to the relationship would it be for the premed to ask her advisor if they are outsourcing their letter writing to a temp worker ghostwriter? And by the way, what would the advisor say if your premed had a ghostwriter draft their personal statement to medical school, even if your premed told the writer what needed to go into it and then reviewed it before it was sent to the medical schools? How is one of these ethically better or worse than the other?

The Prehealth Advising Program

Undergraduate prehealth advising programs can often provide more resources for your premed than just conversations with the advisor and the committee letter. Note that some schools have neither, and many schools do not offer committee letters. The prehealth advising office maintains informational websites, offers regular topical briefings, brings medical school admissions officers to campus, and assembles panels of postbac programs and recent alumni in medical school. They usually publish an email newsletter alerting students to summer and post-graduate opportunities. Often the prehealth advisor is the staff coordinator of the premed club or clubs on campus. Coordinating all of this takes up a large chunk of her time during the academic year.

The most effective premed advisors push factual information out through these many info-vehicles. That means that they can use their one-on-one time for truly individualized concerns. It's frustrating for the advising office staff when applicants have clearly not read and processed the information they send them through email and newsletters, so it's good to remind your premed to do this. Time alone with the premed advisor is all too similar to the precious time you get alone with your doctor in her office. Be prepared, write down a list of issues and questions and bring them to the conversation. You can teach these skills to your premed so they get the advising they need and also earn the respect of the advisor by asking her questions that require her to tailor her facts to your premed's situation. At my website, you can find a list of good questions to ask the advisor.

At schools that offer advisor-managed committee letter processes, it is imperative for them to build a relationship with the advisor over the years. It also helps to have a trusting relationship so the advisor is comfortable admitting that they do not know the answer to a question. Coach your premed to create trust with the advisor over time. Additionally, the premed may need to sort out something confidential with the advisor and need to trust them not to share it. Often premeds do not share anything they really need to talk over because they assume, fear or suspect that the advisor will put it in their committee letter. They need to seek guidance when they need it, and then believe the advisor when she assures them that she will not share that in their letter or to others.

Advocacy for Your Applicant

Often applicants and their parents think that the institutional premed or prehealth advisor at the undergraduate school or postbac program is an ideal influencer and advocate. You can encourage your premed to consider this assumption long in advance by establishing a meaningful, respectful and reciprocal relationship with the advisor throughout college. Yes, it is the advisor's job to guide all applicants, but it is much more motivating for them to work with someone whom they know and understand, whose situation they fully appreciate. This is not to say that advisors play favorites, but relationships do matter. Your premed needs to think about this before the summer moment that they need and seek the advisor's help.

While advisors sometimes are good advocates at medical schools, it's difficult, if not impossible, for them to be all things to all people. And in fact, some advisors are specifically prohibited by their institutions from advocating on behalf of individual students. When I worked at Cornell, we had over 400 AMCAS applicants annually. Naturally, many applied to the New York state schools, and there were over 300 applicants from our school annually to Weill Cornell Medicine and over 200 to Boston University School of Medicine. Cornell is a feeder to many popular medical schools. When their institution is a feeder school, college advisors have to show a lot of discipline and discretion in their advocacy. The Drexel University undergraduate advisor can't send a list of 125 applicants to her colleague at the medical school asking that they all get a close review, and expect that to matter to the admissions officers. This is why institutional premed advisors are not good choices for advocacy in general. It's better to seek advocacy in general from someone who isn't allegiant to so many applicants, which is where principal investigators (PIs) in research labs can play an important role, as we write about in a later chapter on networking.

Medical schools get a lot of applicants. More than a handful get over 10,000 completed applications for 100 spots. Because of this, medical school admissions committees do ask the prehealth advisors at undergraduate schools for this kind of help. At joint meetings, they publicly request advisors to please bring to their attention an applicant they may have overlooked who might be a good fit for that school. Premed advisors love the opportunity, theoretically, to call an admissions dean and say: Look at my student! Pick my Ace of Hearts from your massive deck and give her a shot at acceptance!

I can elucidate two reasons why deans make this request. The first is that they too feel overwhelmed by the task of selection and want to acknowledge publicly that subjectivity plays a role in it. The second is that they believe that there are gem applicants out there and they know that their process just doesn't have the discernment to find them reliably. The reason why their well-intentioned invitation is actually very hard to accept is simple. Premed advisors want their applicants to get into medical school. Usually they support multiple applicants to every school. How does one choose from 5 or 50 applicants to the same medical school just who is the gem to advocate for? The advisor doesn't know them all equally well, but when it comes between an applicant for whom that medical school might be their only chance, and the student who served as the advisor's peer advisor in her office and volunteered to deliver groceries to her shut-in parents during the coronavirus, whom will she advocate for? It's really difficult to choose.

Some applicants are comfortable asking their advisors to advocate at schools they hope to attend; others are not. Just because they ask does not obligate the advisor to help them out. The advisor may need to reconcile many competing agendas. The advisor may or may not see the applicant requesting their advocacy as a good fit for that school. Thus she will justifiably conclude that her advocacy will go nowhere and she will be reluctant to use her chance to help on an endeavor that seems off from the beginning. Ten or twenty other applicants may also be asking the advisor for the same advocacy. At the same time, the advisor has applicants who aren't getting interviews and applicants who are. If you have two applicants, one with three interviews and the other with none, which would you give the edge to in your advocacy if you could not advocate at the same school for both? The advisor's reasoning cannot be shared with advisees most of the time. It's just too hard to tell—and too hard to hear—in the climate of an intense admissions cycle.

Most advisors only advocate on the basis of two criteria: Will you definitely go to that school if I advocate for you? Prove it to me before I go out on a limb for you. Second, do you really need my advocacy? Why should I spend it on someone who prefers Medical School X to the others where you have been admitted?

If an applicant has no interview invitations in January, or only waitlists in April, and is a great applicant, then the premed advisor might reach out. But in that case, is she really recommending a hand-selected ideal fit applicant for Medical School X? Not likely. The dean will see this, and it may lower the credibility of the premed advisor and their future advocacy.

Despite the conflicts, tensions and judgments that the premed advisor needs to make regarding advocating, when it comes right down to it, that phone call is only rarely going to make a difference. Advisors are better at advocating for interviews than anything else. Sometimes they can help at the tail end of waitlist season. Advisors don't "place" or get people into medical school. Advisors listen, support and offer facts tailored to the premed's situation. It's worth consulting them throughout the cycle. Some advisors can offer outstanding advice on networking, just when the premed needs it most, even if they can't do the advocacy themselves. They can connect undergraduates with alumni studying at the medical schools where they are applying. They can brainstorm with the advisee about who could serve as their letter of recommendation writers, and later in the cycle, who on the faculty might be in a position to reach out to medical schools. Sometimes the PI or head of the applicant's research lab can effectively advocate with people they know at the school. At schools the undergraduate institution feeds to, the advisor may know who to call and how best to reach that person. She may know what they like to hear from advocates.

Private Medical School Admissions Advisors

On an institutional basis, universities hire people who know how to find accurate factual information about their own internal workings (the courses, curriculum, student clubs, offices like Career Services and how to use them) as well as external sources of facts and opportunities, and to dispense it with discretion. This generally limits advisors to sharing facts that are tailored to an individual advisee's situation. It is logical for the applicant to expect the advisor to "know" her, but that expectation may be unrealistic, depending on the advisor's workload.

To do "best practice" advising, in my view, the advisor is responsible for truly knowing the applicant and how their many experiences, attributes, competencies and metrics, to use the trade lingo, express their suitability for a life in medicine from the perspective of the committees on admissions. This responsibility extends to understanding the applicant's narrative and how to unfurl it, staging the admissions process as it unfolds by providing details in the optimal format (primary, secondary, interview, updates), by forging with the applicant an individualized timeline, and reviewing everything the advisee will submit to medical schools from this knowing perspective. The advisor serves other roles, in comforting and counseling the applicant, as well as strategizing on developments in the narrative and setbacks in the process. The medical school admissions process can be bruising. When this quality of advising cannot be provided institutionally, it can be sought through a private advising relationship.

In 2013, I left my university prehealth advising job and, at the urging of several then-current applicants, decided to offer premed advising independently. As a career move, it was equal parts scary and fascinating to step outside of the container of the academic institution and into the unknown. I had some humble pie to digest because, like most institutional prehealth advisors, I had always been faintly suspicious of the motives, skills and orientation of the few private advisors I had come across. Later, I realized that actually, I was a little envious of the independent advisor's ability to really significantly help their applicants, whereas I was constrained in so many ways, both subtle (siloed off in the prehealth advising office) and blatant (not enough time!) in my desire to use all that I had learned to guide students effectively. Students tend to hide from their institutional premed advisor the fact that they are working privately with another advisor because of that climate of mistrust, suspicion and envy.

The simple truth is that both institutional and independent premed advisors can be incurious, and poorly informed. They can be dream crushers or oblivious to the realities of this competitive process. They can be all those things, some of those things or none of those things. The issue becomes, how to discern if your institutional premed advisor can meet your needs, or, if you need additional guidance, how to choose the best independent premed advisor for you. I have a lot of respect for certain institutional advisors and certain independent ones.

I can categorize the different independent advisors, name some whom I think premeds should talk with in their search for their own and give you some good questions to ask them. I will let you know the questions I am most often asked when people are comparing advisors and give you some even better ones to ask. I will also share my own independent advising system, how I have grown it, and why we think the particular methodologic approach and tools that we offer optimizes all premed's chances to get into schools where they can prosper and develop as physicians, professionals and compassionate human beings.

Independent advising is an additional investment in an already expensive process. I am writing this book in the hope that families who cannot afford my services, or those who cannot see the value in them, will have the nuanced information they need to serve as their own premed's advisor. **Maybe you are the one to help me realize my next dream: developing an online parents-of-premeds community where we can work together on behalf of all applicants equitably.**

Independent advisors differ in background in some major ways. Their experiential history and credentials give clues to how helpful they may be as guides for you and your premed. Some are doctors, others come from the wild west of test prep and want to help in a broader capacity, and some come from the world that hatched me: university prehealth advising. The doctors tout their experience of having been through the admissions cycle and medical school, and having many friends and colleagues who may have inside experience from being on an admissions committee. Sometimes a doctor will spend their last years of employment doing premed advising privately, as a form of giving back in retirement. Physician advisors frequently advertise themselves and their experience as the gold standard in advising, and criticize the institutional prehealth advisor, as in this excerpt from Jessica Freedman, MD's guide:

...only someone who has actually worked for an extended time on a medical school faculty and who understands what goes on behind the scenes in a medical school admissions office can offer a nuanced understanding of what it takes to be accepted. Premedical advisors are often underinformed and overwhelmed... There is no formal training for becoming an undergraduate premed advisor...

Dr. Freedman goes on to give several examples of how she saved the day and the cycle for these victims of faithless and dream-crushing, rigid institutional advisors, and concludes:

The premed advisors with whom these applicants worked were not malicious, but...most likely...overwhelmed with large numbers of students, not familiar with the medical school admissions process, or did not fully understand what the admissions committees are seeking. The premed advisors also might not have had enough time to really get to know these applicants on more than a superficial level...[13]

The comment about formal training is curious, since MDs-turned advisors do not have any formal training in the work either. They are guided by their experience, Q&A with people they know, their advisees' experience, and the same source you and your premed will use: the internet search engine. Of the doctors, there are those still in medical training who, having been asked to mentor younger students, feel like they deserve to monetize their knowledge, and they become independent advisors. Sometimes doctors just get very interested in medical school admissions and decide to make it their main occupation.

As a premed advisor, I hope that everyone I am guiding into medical school actually participates in the physician workforce

---

13 Freedman, Jessica MD. The Mededits Guide to Medical School Admissions, p. 13-14, published 12/11/18 by MedEdits Publishing

for at least awhile. I always wonder why doctors want to be premed advisors, but sometimes I get good answers for this. Ryan Gray, MD, who operates a virtual megaphone for medical school admissions through his website, app for applicants, and books, is a great example. Ryan is a lifelong learner, who consults with many significant players in the medical school admissions world through his podcast series. Ryan's motto is "collaboration, not competition," a critical message in the hyper-competitive world of medical school admissions. Ryan loves advising.

Institutional premed advisors belong to professional organizations that offer meetings, conferences and school visits on a national, regional and local level. Medical school admissions officers host and present at these meetings, and this is the formal professional development arm of premedical advising. The main organization is the National Association of Advisors to the Health Professions (NAAHP.org) and the less-specialized one, also a player, is the Independent Educational Consultants Association (IECAonline.com).

Sometimes a medical school admissions director, a non-MD staff position, will leave their work or moonlight in medical school admissions. Depending on their level of collegiality with other admissions directors and their session attendance at NAAHP conferences and the AAMCs Group on Student Affairs (GSA) meetings, they will have a broad understanding of admissions. A person who has sat on medical school admissions committees for one school knows a lot about that school, just like you know a lot about your premed, but you need to probe to learn if such an advisor is going to be able to advise with specificity about admissions nuances at many schools. Some independent advisors have served as institutional premed advisors and admissions officers. This is a strong credential indeed. These advisors have gained a lot of perspective on the process and have returned to what they love, advising a few people well. Sylvia Robertson is a good example of this.

The advisors who come to medical school admissions consulting from the test prep or pre-college advising world are usually entrepreneurial and have a sincere helping orientation. They have lived and worked outside of academia and have a healthy disdain for the status quo. The good ones have read everything they could get their hands on and advise from that knowledge bank. They tend to look outside the box for innovative strategies to guide their applicants. These advisors tend to be irreverent and fun to work with. They won't let your premed get stuck worrying about a lot of stuff that seems irrelevant to the big trajectory, like whether thank you notes should be sent via email attachment or in the body of the email. The absolute best example of a keenly attuned, caring and well-tooled advising company in this mold is Passport Admissions, founded by Rob Humbracht, its CEO. His well-honed and time-tested approach works for his many applicants.

By well-tooled, I refer you to his side site, The Savvy Premed, where you can find the best medical school database on the internet. Rob is a deeply altruistic person, who loves to learn new things, whose confidence in his applicants is unshakeable, and whose fountain of good nature and wit has dried up his applicants' tears on many occasions. He is an advisor you can trust.

The Mentoring Alliance

Advisors like me, with an institutional prehealth advising background, lack the personal experience of going through medical school and residency and becoming practicing medical doctors. They often come from higher ed counseling backgrounds, from pre-professional career services offices and for one reason or another, decide to work independently. My reasons for developing an independent advising practice were that, first, my university and I needed to part ways. I was not content to have my professional advising consist of big-group, transactional advising and I wanted to increase our student's success rate (hovering around 55-60%), which I considered pathetic with respect to the quality of our outstanding premeds. I wanted to revolutionize our advising office, making outcomes better, and I wanted to strengthen our relationships with stakeholders outside of our school by cultivating strong collegial relationships with medical schools.

My supervisor did not share these goals and decided she did not want to support them. One advisor would be enough for 2,000 advisees and they could make it work, and so I was pushed out. I want to be candid here and say it wasn't mutual. Several applicants maintained their relationships with me after I left, explaining the world of independent advising to me, and how they had benefited from it.

I decided to work with applicants privately and formed The Mentoring Alliance.[14] It's my goal to see all my applicants go on to mentor and support the applicants in the current admissions cycle while they are training in medical school and beyond. Since I began in 2013, I have been joined by a handful of institutional advisors and an admissions dean. We have developed a system that contains all the requisite features: selecting schools, primary application essay review, secondary essay review, interview preparation, and follow-up action consulting for waitlists. In addition, each applicant who works with us completes a strengths assessment and an extensive questionnaire, which are then discussed during a session of about two hours with two advisors, where we comb through their candidacy in depth, resulting in a report that describes comprehensively the applicant's narrative for medical school admissions.

We call this the narrative build. It allows applicants to plan ahead and to use each of the application essays they write and their interviews to support and strengthen the medical school's view of them as complete applicants who are ready, willing, and able to study medicine and who have the mind, heart, and soul of a physician. By the time we have completed the narrative build, our applicants have responded thoughtfully to most of the questions they will have to answer over the next 18 months, and we know

---

14 www.premedadvisor.com

each other very well. They have experienced an assessment of their candidacy from two contrasting perspectives, and they have a concrete list of what they must develop over the ensuing year to strengthen and distinguish themselves as applicants. And they have someone to text and call whenever an issue or question arises.

How to Choose an Independent Advisor

In order to choose the best premed advisor for you and your premed, you should discuss all the things you and they wished their institutional advisor could have provided, if she had the time, knowledge and resources to do so. Here are some additional considerations.

- Do you want to be part of this process and have access to the advisor?
- Does your premed need work on self-assessment of their candidacy?
- Does your premed thrive from professional consultation, feedback and editing on their writing?
- Does your premed learn best and gain confidence from consulting books on how to write the personal statement and other facets of advising? Will they suffice as resources?
- Does your premed thrive from connection with a personal human guide?
- Is your premed able to embody their professional presentation of self?
- Do you both just feel lost and would like some well-informed human company on this journey?

Imagine what you need and what you hope for in terms of help. How do you see that human touch helping you and your premed accomplish this step of the dream—getting into medical school? Write it all down, agree to disagree as you consider these questions together.

When I conduct these orientation sessions, I like the applicant to come as if it was an advising session and I am the advisor. I don't want to evaluate the candidacy by reviewing a transcript and resume before we talk, but I do want to start by responding to the applicant's authentic advising questions, so the applicant gets a feel for my professional ability. Then, if I am asked to, I will go over the elements of the cycle and how we work through the advising relationship for each element. I am then curious to know what the applicant feels they will need from an advisor.

I am happy on request to conduct these sessions over video and record them so the applicant can share the conversation with their parents or sponsors. I am also happy to include the parents/sponsors in this conversation or a subsequent one. Based on our conversation, I will sometimes recommend and refer the applicant to other independent advisors, including those who collaborate under my umbrella, The Mentoring Alliance.

Each advisor and advising company offers distinct methods and should specify the scope of contact. It is yours to choose what is best for you. For example, many packages specify a limit on the number of drafts of a particular essay that will be reviewed.

Some critical interpersonal things for your applicant to observe in the initial meeting include:

- Do you feel that you have the full and focused attention of the advisor?
- Do you feel listened to, well and fully?
- Do you sense that this person can—and wants to—help you build and sustain your confidence in your chances throughout the admissions cycle?
- When you get feedback from this person on ways to build a stronger candidacy, does it feel negative, hurtful or dismissive? Or does it feel collaborative and kind?
- Would you act on the advice this person gives?
- Are you speaking with the person who will do most of the advising? How does referral work and will you have

the opportunity to speak with a different advisor before you commit to working together?

Since you don't get to choose your college advisor, make sure you do choose your medical school admissions consultant with clear intention about what you need and what you want. Everybody is nice, friendly and accommodating on the initial call, so remember that it's okay to dig a bit before you commit.

Other Sources of Guidance and Support

Websites

The internet is a vast resource of boilerplate information on medical school admissions and we all know we must practice discernment in taking the information we find there to heart. Often, we find ourselves dismissing the information at first glance, but then letting it reside in our subconscious, adding to our stress and uncertainty. This is particularly true for your premed, who wonders: Do I really need to have that whatever thing—score, experience, course—to get into medical school? They know that they don't, but their subconscious entertains itself by dwelling in uncertainty about it. When this happens, it's good to check in with a trusted advisor. It's even better for your premed to trust themselves, be who they are, and have confidence in their skills, experiences and accomplishments.

A word of advice for you and your premed: Don't believe everything you read, don't believe everything you hear, don't waste your time trying to glean real information from studentdoctor.net (SDN) and its copycat sites. My favorite line in the whole universe of SDN is this: "It's Okay to Not Know Everything." That post is actually the title of a piece about the firehose of the first year medical school curriculum, but it's even more suitable as a premed affirmation. Hold onto it; maybe even put it on the refrigerator, because there will be times when your best response to your premed's lament, or even their unanswered question is: *It's okay not to know everything, darling.*

Most important of all: Don't believe everything you think; and remind your premed not to believe everything she thinks, after you have gone ahead and trolled the internet. Don't either of you spend the time waiting to get into medical school assessing false or incomplete claims about the likelihood of it happening or not.

Throughout the admissions cycle, how it all works and how your premed is faring is going to be on your mind. If you consider the approximate 75,000 people (and just think of the number of friends and relatives per applicant!) who are actively in the admissions cycle for medical, dental and other schools at one time, it's truly amazing how much intelligent headspace is being wasted on worry, stress, as well as discounting received wisdom and unsolicited advice from people who like to weigh in on the process. Try to exercise discipline and think about more interesting things. It's fine to let yourself be interrogated and advised at social gatherings where people mean well, but there are some situations where you should be a commando warrior about such matters.

If your premed is already doubting himself or feeling particularly worried, they need to work on the self-talk in and of itself, before they take in more input from family and friends. Think of negative self-talk as a smoldering fire, and input related to the worry as fuel and oxygen to flame that fire. If you don't smother that fire before you add more to it, like any fire, it can get out of your control and more seasoned professionals will be needed to help extinguish that negative mentation.

MSAR, NAAHP Volunteers

I want to recommend you to experts and the true authorities you can find in the internet jungle. The National Association of Advisors to the Health Professions (NAAHP) has volunteer advisors who you can connect with for answers to your questions. The AAMC publishes an online database, called the MSAR, which you have to purchase, but which contains a treasure trove of information on each school. At this writing, there is a, perhaps, even better database at savvypremed.com, a resource you will find invaluable.

Life Coaches, Therapists, Mentors and Spiritual Counselors

Finally, remember that advisors are not the only helping professionals who can guide you and your premed through the admissions process. It's really hard to define the role of an advisor, because it depends so much on the relationships that they build with their advisees, as well as their training and intentions for advising.

Confidence, self-worth and a strong positive expression of personal affect are critical to both wellness and success for premeds. Many touch points can cause these to waver in the healthiest person. When they do, it may be good to call in a few other professionals. As the parent of a premed, it's your responsibility to be in such good communication with your premed that you see this happening at least as soon as they do, but even better, before.

The MCAT is no SAT, it's like no college final exam, and the score on the MCAT never matters more than when the premed is studying for it and hoping for a high score. The combination of tedium and tension in the marathon of preparing for the MCAT can be a volatile mix. The day the score comes can be devastating or throw a premed into existential uncertainty, as can waiting up to six months for the college prehealth office to send out the committee letter. Waiting again, for over half a year, to hear from medical schools is particularly tough for arguably the most driven and achievement-oriented (by necessity, if not nature) kind of person, your premed. When neither you, nor the advisor, nor anyone else in their circle of trust can give the premed what they needs, consider hiring a life coach or therapist.

The reason I think life coaches are worth considering is because they work on a different level than therapists. A life coach takes you from being okay, to setting your intentions to be great. In general, a therapist shows you the way out of your pit of despair and gives you new coping tools. Both these professionals are supportive, but sometimes premeds feel pathologized at the therapist's office. When they are going through normal human highs and lows, sometimes a life coach can help them get back on track in a positive direction in pursuing their future goals.

It may serve your premed—and your own worried suspicions—to consult a therapist for assessment, to make sure there are no underlying signs of symptoms of mental illness. If your premed is just down and drained, a life coach can help them right their mood, self-efficacy and confidence for facing the next round of their journey to medical school.

9 Learning Issues, Accommodations and Obstacles

Because medical schools are able to select from a group of people with very high GPA's, students always feel a deep obligation, even a compulsion, to get the A. Nothing less will do. However this is not necessarily true. In the real world, if a person has half As and half Bs, that gives them a GPA of 3.5. Even though some medical schools have average GPAs for their matriculants of 3.6, 3.7, 3.8 and 3.9, in general, if a person has over a 3.6 (which is a few more As than Bs), they have every reason to think that they can become medical doctors and study at an American school.

One of the principal differences between secondary and higher education, which drives adjustment issues among students, is that in higher education, the teacher is essentially no longer responsible for the student's learning—the student is 100% accountable for their own mastery. In higher education, it is well-established that faculty are rewarded far more consistently for scholarly output, including scientific research than for their teaching. What an unfortunate confluence of systemic factors! Just when their teachers are disincentivized to teach by the system that recruits, hires and compensates them, the students are expected to become wholly responsible for their own learning! No wonder we as advisors see such a sad smear of Cs in our former top-10%-of-the-class, first year college students.

Some professors are great teachers in terms of classroom showmanship and giving students an enjoyable classroom or lecture hall experience, and some just aren't. Some are really weak teachers who don't enjoy the role and are forced into it. Some professors don't try at all to design their lectures to accommodate learning styles, and privately may consider accommodation requests from the Office of Accessibility Resources to be unreasonable. They even sometimes claim that legally mandated accommodations are introducing unfairness into their evaluation model. I know this is also true in high school, but in college the consequences for someone who wants to go into medical school are much more severe, so it is important for students to understand how they learn best and how to cope with and compensate for any learning issues they experience.

Learning Issues

It is important for parents to notice in high school if they can detect a discrepancy between classroom performance and standardized test scores. When there is a large discrepancy, something is off. It could be the quality of instruction and assessment at the school. But it could also be a sign of a neurodivergent way of learning on the part of your child. Learning difference testing is expensive but may be covered through health insurance. It is important to lay down the documentation before entering college because if something is found, it can help your child to show their intelligence and potential accurately, both in college and when the MCAT, GRE, GMAT or other standardized exam rolls around.

In making this recommendation, I sense the scepter of hovercraft parenting arising. Many of us have read accounts in the media of parents who paid learning specialists to fabricate learning difference test results for their children so they could take exams in quiet rooms with relaxed time constraints. We really can't worry if people will think of us in this stereotypical and stigmatizing way. And your student will not be stigmatized for any disability that is detected and assessed. Such practices are illegal and enforced.

I counseled an applicant with aggravated and well-documented learning disabilities who was dismissed from a Caribbean medical school after failing to pass an important test for the second time. She was not granted the accommodations she needed for the exams. The applicant was severely dyslexic and the accommodation was to be able to ask the proctor to read the question aloud. She failed by just a few points to pass a pathology multiple choice exam where the names of terms were multisyllabic and long. The school would not allow the human proctor to read the items to her. The school had been accredited by the US government to qualify its students for federal loans. The medical student's family hired a lawyer who specialized in legally mandated accommodations.

The lawyer pointed out to the medical school administration that if they were reported to the Department of Education for failing to provide legally mandated accommodations to any student, they would lose their main source of funding: US guaranteed loans, which nearly all their students used to finance their medical education. The school quickly reinstated my applicant and re-administered the test with proper accommodations. She successfully passed it and she is now a practicing psychiatrist in the United States.

Accommodations

Students with learning disabilities need to take a very careful approach to curriculum planning, especially in terms of not overloading their academic schedules. Many premed prerequisite science courses are taught by lecturing large groups of students, and are often tested with multiple choice exams that can be easily graded and where students can be assessed by a simple score in terms of their deviation from the mean (also known as being graded on a curve). This is a very difficult way for students who have learning disabilities to be graded. The only accommodations that can be provided are either to take the test in a private room with no distractions, or to be given extra time (time and a half or double time). These types of cookie cutter accommodations don't necessarily compensate for individual learning differences.

Students who don't have documented learning disabilities, but who know they study better with more time or in quiet rooms or with fewer people can really benefit from talking to their faculty about that and choosing courses that provide the most conducive learning environment. It is worth asserting themselves and asking for what they need.

Students with accommodations in high school often want to drop their accommodations in college because they either think that they have overcome their learning disabilities through training in secondary or primary school, or they don't want to be stigmatized. Every student who has accommodations is best served by holding on to them and continually keeping strong documentation of receiving them.

Somewhere after sophomore year, student attention will turn to taking the Medical College Admissions Test (MCAT). The MCAT Accommodations Service takes applications for accommodations and grants such accommodations. As mentioned earlier, if a student stopped asking for and receiving accommodations during college, it can be really hard to get accommodations for the MCAT. In medical school, residency and licensing renewal, people face lots and lots of standardized testing and those tests are even harder to gain accommodations for. This is why it's important for parents to insist on letting go of any concern regarding stigma at being labeled as a person who needs testing accommodations. It is the job of the parent to make sure that any child with any kind of learning difference, even while they are encouraged to compensate and move beyond them as much as possible, should be tested every couple years and continue to apply for, seek and accept accommodations, so when they get to the point where they are taking extremely high stake examinations, they have the support they need to take the test on their own terms.

I look forward to the day when all students get choices about how much time and what testing environment they want and need. The only thing preventing that is the economics of higher education, which improves its own bottom line, and saves their faculty time for their research, through grading systems based on machine graded and statistically analyzed multiple choice exams.

Some medical schools will grant students accommodations for any reason at all. They will allow any student who requests it to take an exam over a longer time period than scheduled, or in a quiet and comfortable space. They trust their students.

Other Obstacles: Anxiety-Provoking Unexpected Events

Sometimes the worst happens and your student's requests for accommodation, for whatever reason, may not be heeded. This may be due to a poorly informed test proctor, busy professor or just lack of time, concern or care on the part of the person or institution administering the test. When this happens, it can provide additional stress for a student who also suffers from anxiety. Additional creative strategic work may be needed to assure that your student gets the accommodations they deserve. Don't give up. It's important to creatively advocate for your student to get the resources they need.

One of my applicants, Morgan, received extra time accommodations on the MCAT because of his documented anxiety. As is well known, anxiety sucks up a person's cognitive resources. When he felt he was becoming anxious, he was allowed to ask that the test be suspended for a 15 min break. Because the MCAT is 7.5 hours long, accommodations for extra time dictate that the test be administered over two days. In Morgan's case, he took the first half of the exam on a Saturday, and at the end of the first day of the exam, he was informed by the proctor that he could not complete the exam the next day. He was not given a reason why. This determination was put to him in such a perfunctory way that he actually couldn't believe it was true. He left the exam center and called the MCAT help line dozens of times that evening and night. Because it was Saturday night, he didn't get a response. Finally, late Saturday night, someone who did not identify if they were an employee of the testing center or of MCAT called Morgan to tell him not to report the next day, and that because of technological issues, he would have to reschedule the exam and retake the whole thing.

It's hard to convey how distressing something like this is for a student at the time it is happening. Morgan had planned, studied and scheduled the exam so it would be done before he went back to school, and now he would have to jockey online for MCAT test dates while attending school, and take the test in mid-semester. Luckily, Morgan was living at home and his parents were able to completely turn themselves over to being with him.

They consulted with me and I fortunately had the email address of the person at AAMC who supervises the MCAT, whom I could write to and ask for help. I only had that email address because I admired something this administrator said at a meeting I attended and went up to thank her for what I had learned from her, at the end of her presentation. She gave me her business card, which I kept. After I wrote to the administrator, she kept me abreast of her work to remedy the situation and I was able to update the parents so they could appease the terrible anxiety the student was experiencing. In the end, Morgan did retake the test, got his score and moved on in life. It's worth pulling all your resources together to get your students the accommodations they deserve. Sometimes it does take a village to remedy a problem.

One more note: When a premed is prone to anxiety and depression, it's important for them to have a clearly delineated strategy for working their way through their "stuff" before it becomes unmanageable. Parents, life coaches and therapists all have the ability to sit with the premed and draw up a guide for navigating it, no matter what arises. It's important for the parent to be involved because you know the triggers and you care the most. It becomes a kind of pre-college agreement for when it's okay for you to intervene, advocate and help fish them out of the broiling waters of misery.

10 Outside the Classroom: Choosing Extracurriculars

While applicants to medical school must focus time and attention on their academics, at least half of the personal growth they will need to demonstrate in their application will come from experiences outside of the classroom.

Service

The most important activity premeds can engage in is serving others in community or clinical settings, particularly in a way that aligns with the premed's own passions and strengths. In high school, it makes sense for a premed to engage in service activities with a parent, friend, or peer group. It's not something she should do by herself. It helps to reflect and grow from the experience if you do it with someone else. When premeds serve alongside their family, it helps them embody their family values. When asked to reflect on how their commitment to service developed, a lot of premeds write about their parents instilling the value of service to their community when they were growing up.

The service activities your premed engages in need to make sense in terms of their emerging understanding of what turns them on and what turns them off, or if you will, what energizes them and what drains them. If they participate in service that energizes them, they are a lot more likely to learn important things, network with people who will become mentors, and enjoy the activity enough to show an ongoing commitment. High school premeds who engage in service have an early opportunity to make a difference, develop leadership skills, and clarify their passion for helping others. If you join a service activity based on the needs of a family member (e.g., my sister has autism, grandma has dementia), your child sees a broader range of the same issue, develops a deep sense of empathy for others, and can come back and help their own family; it makes for a really good narrative.

In high school and college, premeds who want to be doctors should serve populations in need—older adults, people in nursing homes or hospice, socioeconomically disadvantaged populations. If they find the opportunity to be of service in a clinical or community health setting, they will grow from relationships with diverse community members and from observing the skills and strategies of doctors and other health professionals. These premeds have a realistic view of the medical profession, which is important to medical schools.

A lot of premeds will volunteer in pediatric hospitals but only play with pediatric patients in the playroom. The premed may think, "I love kids, I loved my pediatrician: I'll be a pediatrician." But they may not have actually spent time with the kids who are very sick and observed the ups and downs of the nurses and physicians who care for them. The experience of going to your pediatrician whom you love is very different from seeing that pediatrician burnt out, infected a hundred times from the colds and flus that showed up in the office, and enduring fatigue when they are behind the scenes. It's important that when the premed emerges from high school, they've seen suffering and know that they still want to be a doctor; this clarity will motivate them when they get to the rigorous academics and experience obstacles in college.

There are also many ways to engage in service remotely, such as providing computer or phone support, or emotional companionship, to older adults in nursing homes or alone at home.

Tutoring

Tutoring is a great service activity because it allows premeds to give back what they know to others and to complete the loop of teaching and learning reciprocity. It also gives them confidence, teaches them about mental health, and is an opportunity for them to practice how to communicate in an agile way. The final stage of mastery is being able to teach others. Tutoring or TAing (being a teaching assistant for a professor) allows the premed to reinforce their own learning, which is important if they are tutoring subjects they've learned in class that will be on the MCAT. Tutoring allows premeds to immerse themselves to some degree in other people's family experiences and learning challenges—it develops empathy and cultural competence. In addition to peer-to-peer academic tutoring and TAing, your premed can consider volunteering for a non-profit like Masteryhour.org (where college students can volunteer to tutor math to underserved children), Big Brothers Big Sisters of America, or tutoring a foreign language independently. There are also opportunities to teach foreign students English or help younger students in under-funded schools with their college applications.

College Clubs: Passion and Leadership

In college, it's important that premeds don't join particular clubs just because older friends who are leaders need more bodies in the room. Choices should not be predicated on a friend wanting them to do it and looping them in—they must really want to do it. Your premed can try different clubs in college to get a sense for what interests them and find a community they can invest in, but it is best for them to eventually settle on one or a few groups and invest a couple years into that activity.

Most clubs have a pathway to leadership. Sometimes the pathway is very political. Sometimes nobody wants to run the club and the path to leadership is based on whoever doesn't refuse to do it.

People need to consider that when they join a club. If you run a club where no one wants to be on your e-board, it can be hard to keep that going and have a success story to show for it. On the other hand, if your premed has the leadership, initiative, and passion to build something up and make it better than they found it, that really says something about a person; it's a great thing for a premed to write about in their application and it boosts their sense of confidence and agency. Students need to keep in mind that they, too, have a legacy to leave at any organization they engage with. Legacies are important qualities that are looked for in the screening and selection of medical candidates. The story of leaving something better than you found it is well-aligned with the work of a physician.

Your premed doesn't have to be president, but it is not very compelling to be vice-president, secretary, or treasurer unless they really have the ability to make a difference and do something important for the organization or community. They can create a new role, such as director of partnerships or training, or other important aspect of the club's mission. Your premed needs to examine the pathway to leadership, knowing there are many ways to embody leadership, and to chart out their course.

Founding a Club

Sometimes people think that in order to get into medical school they have to be a founder. They start clubs, which is a good experience because they will begin by establishing relationships with the student assembly, learn to budget, and build a community. However, it is important to see if there are similar clubs before they start—if there are more than two, they can start an umbrella organization to bring sub-communities together. There are often a lot of ethnic clubs in college. If your premed establishes the Pan-Asian Club, they can show a real organizational understanding, and their interest in bringing people together and bridging differences. It provides evidence that they are inclusive and culturally competent.

Sports

Teamwork is one of the competencies that medical schools look for in their applicants, and athletics can be a great way to develop many of the premedical competencies, including cultural competence, social skills, and capacity for improvement. Athletes and people who support athletes often have opportunities to grow as leaders and coaches, and to develop humility, organization, and discipline. One of my applicants transformed his role on the football team from water boy to assistant coach throughout his four years of college. Athletes also have the opportunity to study the human body, learn how to maintain a healthy body and mind, and demonstrate resilience through injuries and setbacks. In an athletic setting, your premed can also find opportunities to shadow or help the trainers and clinical staff.

Experiences with Orthodox Religion

You can look at religious adherence from the scale of very observant to being "spiritual." Applicants who are religiously observant or consider themselves spiritually engaged should reflect regularly in a journal on the insight and personal growth they bring to the practice of medicine and serving others from their religious and spiritual experiences. Here's what I have noticed. Orthodox Jewish applicants, for example, have experienced a really strong interdependent community. They look out for each other and their lives are ruled by strong, but not necessarily rigid, ethical principles. Many religious communities are deeply committed to service and the values derived from religion are an important part of an applicant's narrative.

It is also important that premeds get to know other religions so they can see commonalities that underlie all religions and spiritual practices, and demonstrate cultural competence and inclusivity. In college, people can easily visit student-oriented religious services and the pizza hours that follow. One such premed, Ryan, grew up in a Seventh Day Adventist family. He made friends as soon as he got to college who brought him to their services, luring him with the free food they shared in together during the fellowship hour. When I was interviewing him for his Cornell committee letter, I asked what he had learned from those forays. He replied, "I was brought up to conceive of God as living in the sky above, but now I know that God lies within me." He touched his hand to his heart.

Every religion, and formal atheism included, has much to teach about service and altruism, about community interdependence and safety. All these lessons serve our physicians well in their practice of medicine.

Clinical Engagement

Applicants to medical school absolutely need to have clinical engagement experiences on their applications. Beyond passively shadowing a doctor, clinical engagement indicates that the premed actually has an opportunity to serve in some way, or at the least, to engage with a patient population. One of the most active clinical activities a premed can do is to become EMT-certified (Emergency Medical Technician) and work as a campus EMT to do rescue and response around their campus. The prehealth advising office on campus may have partnerships with health care providers or clinical offices to provide opportunities to their premeds, but it is beneficial for your premed to build their own connections and find opportunities that are related to their interests.

A premed can reach out to the volunteer office at hospitals, or contact local private practices, or ask any medical professional (not just doctors) for an opportunity to shadow or help. It is a good thing for aspiring doctors to gain insight into the work of physical therapists and other allied health professionals because they get a sense of the cycle of healing and the teamwork involved in medical care. Humility is a characteristic medical schools will examine applicants for, and it is essential to gain the understanding that physicians are only one part of the health care team and all members who serve are deserving of respect and have something to teach us from their distinct perspective.

Engagement with a patient population can happen in a nursing home, social services organization, or free clinic. It can strengthen an application to have clinical engagement experience across lifespan and genders, and with medically underserved populations. If your premed identifies with or has a particular dedication to a certain community (e.g., LGBTQIA+, people experiencing homelessness, people with differently abled bodies), it is compelling to see their investment in and service to such a community over time. Some roles your premed might explore include being a patient advocate or helping immigrants and refugees obtain healthcare through a community organization or free clinic.

In the absence of in-person clinical engagement opportunities, a premed can take online clinical education classes, such as the ReelDx-sponsored HEAL Clinical Education Network, which I co-founded with Rob Humbracht during the pandemic when applicants could not gain access to clinical settings. It has proven to be a viable and well-accepted complementary alternative to conventional in-person shadowing. Book clubs and virtual shadowing opportunities are also ways to increase one's understanding of clinical medicine.

Premed Summer Programs

Finally, premedical summer programs are a great way for applicants to gain clinical exposure, improve their understanding of life sciences, chemistry and physics, and develop relationships with mentors. You can find these opportunities through an internet search, the AAMC website, and your premed's undergraduate school's prehealth advising website. Prehealth websites of other colleges are also a great resource, as some schools keep an incredibly vast and up-to-date website directory of opportunities. Many summer programs are designated for socioeconomically disadvantaged premeds and will pay premeds a stipend.

Research

It is worthwhile to find research opportunities in high school because the lab won't give your premed many critical responsibilities, so they can't make beginner mistakes in running experimental protocols. They can mostly observe, clean and stock, and ask questions. If they stay long enough and learn some lab skills, then your premed will have some experience on their resume when they go looking for labs in college, so they have a better chance at getting the positions that interest them.

Research can be bench research in a lab or it can be social research or a literature review. One premed I know, Hannah Fagen, conducted independent research to uncover the history of hospital nurseries and the practice of positioning new babies in their bassinets in rows facing a viewing window so people in the hospital could enjoy looking at them. She published her research in an article subtitled: "The Happiest Place in the Hospital." Another applicant read the entire 906-page Affordable Care Act and summarized it for the physicians in his local hospital. The key to independent research, or really most research, is to find a professor who will sponsor you so you can get course credit and have access to social and financial resources.

Work Experience

Can you believe that some premeds apply to medical school and have no paid work experience they can cite? On the other hand, many applicants need to work in order to support their own living expenses or their family. Admissions officers really appreciate the sense of responsibility and maturity that applicants derive from employment activities. Sometimes premeds get paid for summer research experience. It is a really good idea to be a server or a barista, or work as a dishwasher or furniture mover. That kind of practical, service-oriented job exposes the aspiring physician to the needs and culture of a diversity of employers, coworkers, and customers, and helps premeds develop professionalism, communication skills, social skills, resilience, and humility. Employment brings premeds a deeper understanding of service, economics, and what it means to be a person with less education and less opportunity than they may enjoy.

It can be challenging for students to balance employment with an already dense academic and extracurricular schedule, so why not accomplish simultaneous aims by finding employment in a clinical setting, thus affording both clinical engagement and shadowing opportunities? Premeds can become certified as a phlebotomist, nursing assistant, or doula. Or they can work as a standardized patient or cleaning rooms in a hospital. Any entry-level job that they qualify for is going to impress medical schools through their willingness to serve in that way. One of my applicants trained to be a phlebotomist and then worked shifts at the local hospital while he was a college premed. Now he's a cardiologist.

Capstone Project

Finally, all of these experiences outside of the classroom, and even those in the classroom, are great opportunities for your premed to identify a social or medical problem and develop a capstone project.[15] After they have identified a problem, they can gather information and resources to solve that problem. The solution can be implemented where they work, with an organization, or on their own. The purpose is to demonstrate initiative, service, leadership, commitment, and contribution. The solution should impact a group of people and the results should be shared with a broader community, through a forum or social media. The personal growth and networking relationships your premed nurtures during the capstone project will be invaluable later on in the application process.

---

15 I credit my friend and colleague, Rob Humbracht of Passport Admissions, with hatching the great and profoundly useful idea of the capstone project.

I encourage the development and execution of a capstone project during the period when they are applying. They need not mention the project in their applications, unless it is well-developed and well-underway, but it makes for a great digital media topic to tweet into the universe of medical educators, administrators and admissions people on Twitter. It also makes for a useful update when you want to reconnect after applying and have something to tell the school.

Sometimes a person with a red flag on their application due to an offense committed in college who needs to show that they learned from the transgression, can develop a capstone project to demonstrate this, by helping others avoid the same mistake. One of my applicants who captained a rowdy Division I college team had an alcohol violation. After college, he developed a capstone project to collect and disseminate methods and practices that athletic directors all over the country could use to eradicate the alcohol-soaked cultural ethos of college athletics. He organized thoughtful discussions through a podcast, republished blog posts, and added his own thoughts on the subject. He got into medical school with this demonstration of the extent of his personal development.

Often premeds think that publication of a research article is the only way to show any prominence or impact in the world of science. This is simply no longer true. Anyone with something important to say can develop a capstone project and disseminate their ideas, connect with like-minded mentors and become thought leaders in the twitterverse, on LinkedIn, and in other professional internet venues

11 How Premeds Can Network Effectively

This chapter is about the importance of building a strong mentoring network, which premeds are not directly clued into, much less taught. The importance of knowing how to network and including it in your repertoire as a premed is not at all obvious. It may be the single most invaluable skill that doesn't make it into the premed checklist nor the standard instructions for going through the medical school application process. It's yet another skill to develop, with a very rich payoff, both personally and professionally.

Many observers of the current generation of premeds complain that they keep their eyes on their phones and their ears filled with headphones. When you cut off your vision and your hearing, a counterbalance is needed to make sure you notice, experience and explore the great big world of other people all around you every day. You have to be available to get to know them. This is very important to learning to study collaboratively and to becoming a leader. Medical schools want evidence of both. You can't begin to collaborate or lead with your face in a laptop listening to MCAT questions through your earphones.

Networking Prodigy

I learned the importance of networking from a prodigy of the art. Jeff, a senior when I met him, was a good student, with a 3.7 and a 90 percentile MCAT. He had done everything expected of him as a premed. Extremely well-organized, he brought me a magnificently detailed spreadsheet outlining his game plan for medical school admissions. Jeff hoped I would help him fill in the cells he couldn't. That is a great way to approach and network with your premed advisor.

As I filled in his boxes with the nuances they required, I couldn't help but notice how likeable he was. He presented in a polished and professional way. Every bit of his attire from head to toe, evoked the word "well-groomed" but also "laid back." He was a distinctly compelling applicant, and not by accident. I knew he dressed for our meeting, which took place on campus where few ever thought of dressing to see their premed advisor. Nevertheless, despite the obvious realization that he dressed this way because he wanted to make an impression, I was impressed. Jeff made people feel that they mattered.

In the conversations that took place after we covered his questions, he explained that his undergraduate career was all about meeting people and getting to know them better. He sustained and maintained these relationships, and, when appropriate, learned about his connections' networks. If Jeff thought someone in your network would be good to meet, he asked for an introduction. He knew how to work the concept of "degrees of separation" to minimize the distance between him and people he wanted to know better. As a result, he had a place to stay at every medical school he visited, and he had visited every school where he planned to apply in the summer before his senior year, while he was applying.

On these trips, Jeff had met even more people, visited faculty members in their offices to learn of their research, and gathered extensive information on the quality of student life, the school's culture, what it was proud of about itself, and the little anecdotes that don't make their way far off campus. This allowed Jeff to communicate with schools like they were familiar old friends. I realized that Jeff's parents must have bankrolled this operation, and many applicants just could not afford such travels. But as a son of immigrants, Jeff had learned how to draw people towards him for support, and not to take any of them for granted. Everyone can do more of that. He had developed the mindset that everyone likes and wants to help others, and that we all depend on each other. He was fully committed to being that helpful mentor himself someday.

For Jeff, contacts lead to connections which lead to the life he wants. Because Jeff was so intentional, authentic, and personable, he made it easy for his contacts to be motivated to help him. He did his homework, learning about the interests of the people he would meet. He cared about them and showed that through his open and honest listening. He did not pander or apply lavish flattery. Jeff's ability to work and grow his network brought him access: he knew people with important connections to the opportunities, places, or people he was seeking. He went to Stanford Medical School and did his surgery residency there.

When I write to Jeff, a busy surgeon, he writes back in 24 hours and the first line is an inquiry about how I am doing. Every time I ask him to help one of my premeds learn the ropes for their upcoming interview at Stanford, he invites them to dinner and gives them a place to stay. I learned from Jeff, who took networking to such lengths, that every premed needs to make this part of their modus operandi.

Networking with Professors and PI's

At the 2018 AAMC meeting, I attended a session on networking in medicine designed for physician-scientists, physician faculty and physician administrators. The session introduction said:

Having a knowledgeable and supportive network is critical to the career and personal development of students, residents, and early career academic professionals. Evidence suggests that fewer than half of medical students have a mentor and in some fields of academic medicine, fewer than 20% of faculty had a mentor. Strong networking skills allow individuals to initiate, develop, and maintain rewarding relationships that are meaningful within their desired career paths. A network of mentors can provide guidance on writing and research, information about promotion protocols, or work/life balance.

For those who are underrepresented and women, networking can be a tool to find community and understand institutional culture. Networking as a skill is often left out of undergraduate and graduate medical education and is often met with a certain level of uncertainty. Individuals are hesitant to network because it is often discussed as a one-sided endeavor that doesn't add value for all parties involved. [16]

In college, networking is vital, not optional. Sometimes I wonder why it does not appear on the premed checklist. Maybe because it requires a lot of detail and reinforcement to impart and cannot fit a checklist format. Nevertheless, when your premed is conscientious and engaged in networking, their medical school admissions prospects will undoubtedly increase. The first major networking initiative your premed will undertake in college is recognizing that they depend on others for success, and the relationship is mutual. Your premed will need others to attest to their activities, experiences, and achievements. When they form rich relationships with faculty advisors who oversee the extracurricular engagements they take on, PIs and others who observe them in the lab, coaches of athletic activities, and all the other staff, faculty and community organizations directors and program managers they will interact with, they are building a supportive network that will vouch for them through letters of recommendation. Reference letters are the original networking tool and there are good reasons for why the ancient practice of collecting such letters endures.

---

[16] Smith, S., Bernstein, D., Sánchez, J.P., & Peterson, K. (2018, November 3). Networking Within Academic Medicine [Conference presentation]. Learn Serve Lead 2018: The AAMC Annual Meeting, Austin, TX, United States.

How can your premed build these relationships? Advisors counsel students to attend office hours. That's a start. Giant lecture classes at large universities can make it difficult for your premed to establish true relationships with faculty members. At the university where I worked, students often waited in a line an hour long to have ten minutes of office time with their professor. During the pandemic, there were few face-to-face encounters and we only had video meetings to go on. Nevertheless, applicants who learned to network persisted, and their efforts yielded better letters and effective mentorship opportunities.

There are other ways to build relationships and your premed should look out for them. These include:

- Attending departmental colloquia that the professor of interest is likely to attend.
- Joining clubs on campus that the professor may serve as faculty advisor for.
- Seeking out activities that the faculty member engages in, on campus or off. You may think of that as stalking but it's not, so reframe your mindset. I have often gone to events hoping to deepen a relationship with one person I expect to see (who either never showed up or never got free of the human entanglement surrounding them), only to meet and get to know someone else who became a great connection but had never been on my radar.

It's important—but not required—for your premed to do good work in a research lab for at least one of the upper class years. By good work, I mean coming into the lab consistently curious, dependable, industrious, collaborative and reliable. When premeds work in a research lab, the experience downsizes the impersonal aspect of the university to a small, frequently nurturing, and functional unit. The student becomes known by a few scientists who benefit from his work in their lab. This inestimably valuable learning experience expands their network and increases the chance of getting a good recommendation letter.

Networking with Peers

There are so many interactions every day as students move about campus, not even counting their organized activities: classes, clubs, meals. They need to see other students, particularly more advanced ones, as worth getting to know and becoming connected with. As a premed advisor, I stay in touch with the applicants I have worked with. As they move through medical school, I ask them to share their wisdom with my current group of premeds when they prepare for interviews and arrive on campus. They are happy to do so, not the least because they got that help from the network when they were interviewing. One of the beautiful things about networking is reciprocity. It's a give, give, give and then receive—when you really need it—kind of thing. I call my own advising enterprise The Mentoring Alliance because that is a prime focus of all our work.

Encourage your premed to seek contact information from everyone when they meet them. It may feel weird to ask their peers for this because that is often a flirtatious, pick-up activity, but if that's not the intention, any such illusion can quickly and kindly be dispelled. The critical importance of building that network supersedes any initial discomfort—and it's to the other person's advantage also. Networking is reciprocal; an open loop of giving and receiving. It's very important to ask for their contact information instead of just giving them a business card. Send them a follow-up note within 24 hours. Later, your premed can use this thread to ask for information or introductions so that the contact is reminded of when and how they met. We don't have phone directories anymore and the social media connection systems only work within their domains. Nothing works nearly as well as having your own set of contacts, annotated well to remind you of who the person is and why they matter. The network expands when you remember that each classmate has friends at other schools and families living in different cities, all with their own professional contacts.

Networking with Medical School Students

When the admission cycle begins, it's important for your premed to have connections with students who are now in medical school, so your premed can ask questions about the medical school and how to prepare for interviews.

Networking Exercise for Premeds

Who can I network with? Who have I known through my personal and academic relationships who has a connection with a medical school or physician?

For example: You had a lab partner in college who you worked really well with. Now she is a student at Drexel where you want to apply. Or through LinkedIn you see that her brother is at your first-choice medical school. Find the connection and minimize the degrees of separation until you can meet someone who matters. Then, forge a friendship.

Here are some people to think about to plant and grow the network:

- Family and friend connections
- Pediatricians / dentists / family physicians
- Lab partners, classmates
- Volunteering connections

Building Relationships

Andreas von der Heydt, 2015 author of **The 7 Qualities of Tomorrow's Top Leaders: Successful Leadership in a New Era,** wrote a beautiful chapter on the importance of trust in relationship building of any kind. Because the premed world is often ruthlessly competitive, and students encounter that climate at a tender age when entering college, sometimes they forget how much trust matters.

Today's most selective universities have a huge iceberg submerged under the still waters of academia. Universities may be all about freedom of expression, but we know from the #MeToo movement that, to protect themselves from lawsuits, they turn a blind eye to sexual assault and the drug and alcohol use that often fuels it. In making grading easier for the faculty, whom they want to see producing research publications, they allow grading to be based on multiple choice exams and other mass-processing systems of evaluation. A faculty member who individually tests a student, much less ever once even converses with the students in their classes, is actually rare. The premed course prerequisites have hundreds of students in lectures. Grading is anonymous.

Many of the most high-achieving and successful students at the most competitively selective colleges—whom we like to think of as our best and brightest—illegally buy and sell prescription medications intended for ADHD and other legitimate learning disabilities. They abuse these medications as a shortcut to increased stamina, focus and vitality. In addition, many students cheat, in groups or alone, giving each other and gaining for themselves unfair advantage on exams and other graded assignments. After forty years in the higher education milieu at an Ivy League university, I can confidently assert that the most wily cheaters are never caught. Students who know better than to go down either of those roads realize that they are doing so to their own detriment.

For all these reasons, it's hard for a medical school applicant to prize trust as a core value after undergoing that gauntlet. Students don't turn other students in, for the most part, because the role of informant is one of the loneliest roles on any campus, and also a pretty scary thing to do. This degrades trust as well.

As parents, this issue needs your attention because your premed's trusting relationship with you is inextricably woven into the fabric of your lives together. I know full well that parents sometimes betray the trust their children place in them, and during the teenage years, kids can do the same to their parents. Nevertheless, it is so critical to getting through the path to and within a medical career that you make sure your children talk with you about trust. You need to uphold it for them, exceptions to the rule notwithstanding. I'm suggesting you work this through as a family, and not just so your applicant will feel comfortable and energized in building an effective professional network, obviously. But without fully endorsing the importance of trust in establishing, sustaining and maintaining relationships, the process will be flawed and not reach its potential in launching your applicant into adulthood.

For building lasting and deep relationships, it's important for your premed to understand and learn to express their own motivations and interests, listen closely, openly and honestly to others, and ask their contacts good questions about their work and life.

Another thing to do is to give before needing something in return. On my wall is a card I received totally unexpectedly from a premed, thanking me for a particular interaction we had. Inside, she reflected with gratitude on how my guidance at a tough time led her to deeply accept the truth of those words and how it gave her confidence going forward. When you thank someone in your network, that gesture bonds you to them.

Another gift your premed can give to a staff member (non-faculty) or supervisor at college or in the community is to write a letter to their supervisor noting all the good things the premed has noticed about that person professionally, from their unique perspective. People often ask if email or a social media comment or post is good enough, and of course it is good *enough*, but stationery, cardstock and penmanship go a long way to show consideration, premeditation and the effort to recognize this person. The older the person is, as a general rule, the more they appreciate gestures on paper written by hand.

Networking with Admissions Officers

Your premed will want to go to places where they can meet and talk to medical school admissions officers, so they can get a sense of who your premed really is, face to face.

Places to make physically-based connections:

- College info sessions
- Open houses at medical schools
- Medical career fairs
- Research conferences
- Student Healthcare Professional Associations (e.g., American Medical Student Association, Student National Medical Association)

In-Person Medical School Fairs

Medical school fairs are the single most underutilized venue for getting into medical school. Schools go to great effort to host these events and frequently find them woefully under-attended. Applicants just do not realize what it means to have an opportunity to meet an admissions officer, maybe even the admissions dean, at these events. Every year I make it a priority to attend the AAMC meeting, an event that brings in about 4,000 people who have some relationship to medical education. At these events, I network from sun up to sun down, from the 7:30 am plenary to the 10:00 pm cocktail reception.

One year I noticed that the AAMC was taking advantage of the medical admissions presence at that meeting to hold a medical school fair in person. I told my applicants about it and urged them to show up. They asked me why, how, what to bring, what to say, and I realized how unschooled they were on networking. As I prepared them outside the room where the fair was about to start, two AAMC staff members approached us with several dozen premeds in tow. They asked if these other students could join us. It was then that I knew this work needed to be part of standard premed education.

Everyone who attends a medical school fair has the chance to network with and learn from current medical students, admissions staff, and other premeds. I encourage applicants and premeds to go to every open fair there is, and to write up a debrief to reflect on the interactions they had and what they learned. This is something you could ask your premed to talk with you about. Debriefing is easier with a listener who cares. It's been truly heartening to see how many premeds leave the fair feeling like they are now known at the medical school, and it's also kind of eye-opening how many interviews are generated from these appearances.

If your premed has yet to apply to medical school, the workshops and information at the fair may help them decide which medical disciplines interest them most. The information they gather about particular schools and their application process can help them narrow the list of schools and programs where they will apply.

Medical schools send representatives to fairs in order to recruit a diverse applicant pool. For a premed who has already applied to medical schools and is waiting for an invitation to interview or a letter of acceptance, the fair gives admissions offices their chance to meet them—it's like a pre-interview—they get a sense of your premed or applicant that they can't get from combing through their application.

At spring career fairs, your premed can learn and track each school's mission, what they want in students, and what they are proud of. At fall fairs, such as the AAMC fair, admissions committees are primed to meet and talk to current cycle applicants. The goal for your premed is to get an interview invitation or to be moved from a waitlist to the accepted pool after leaving a good, distinctive and lasting impression. I've seen applicants achieve this goal over and over.

Since then, I have created guiding materials for their attendance at fairs, and I track fairs taking place across the country and find out if they are open to all premeds or limited to the school's own students and alumni.

- Your premed should look good, dress in business casual, and present a neat, clean, and professional demeanor. They can wear a bright colored tie, bowtie, scarf, or accessory to convey vibrancy and distinguish them.

- Bring a business card and a one page summary of their contact information, goal for a career in medicine, and evidence for their core competencies that admissions officers use in holistic review (more information about the medical schools précis, below). These materials can include a professional-looking photograph to help the admissions officers remember them. A photo of your premed in a natural, evenly sunlit outdoor environment, looking relaxed and happy, makes a good impression.
- Thoroughly research the schools they are interested in interacting with and avoid asking the representative questions that could easily be answered by looking at the school's website.
- Carry all of their materials in a professional-looking padfolio or folder, and bring a large, professional bag to carry all of the information they gather.

Premed Précis

The premed version of the resume—which I call a précis to distinguish it from the more business/law oriented resume—provides the experiential evidence and intentions as a function of the AAMC competencies, which are the established attributes that medical schools screen for in their holistic review process. The document also includes a portrait to help medical schools remember the applicant.

Look for the AAMC Core Competencies for Entering Medical Students online to find the competencies that medical schools use in holistic admissions. Pick a subgroup, 7-10 competencies that the applicant has developed, for which they can make the strongest case. As you read through the samples below, notice that each description is about one sentence stating the intention and 1-2 sentences describing the activity that documents the applicant's development of the competency. Here is an example of the précis:

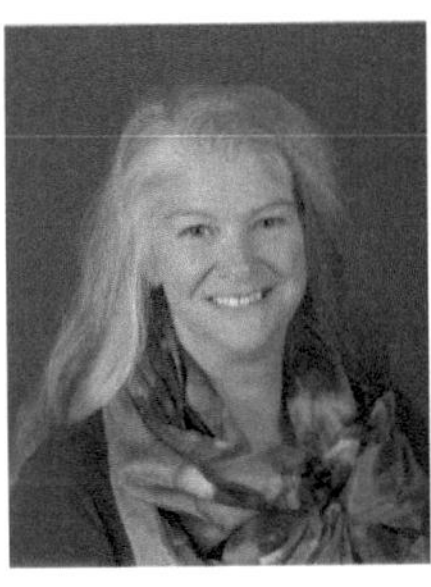

Full Name

University and Graduation Year

Major

Email Address

Summative statement on candidacy: As a future physician, I hope to serve the most under-resourced areas to offer a sense of hope and return dignity to those who need it most. I possess the core competencies that make an effective, compassionate, and dedicated student of medicine.

Service Orientation: I am dedicated to serving my community both locally and globally. I have volunteered at local hospitals for 200+ hours, tutored children in under-resourced schools in Ithaca in STEM fields, organized community events such as hospice center visits or volunteering at local Red Cross shelters, and organized fundraisers raising $3,000+ for various global health causes.

Cultural Competency: My international experiences have opened my eyes to medicine in diverse contexts. I have developed compassion and sensitivity towards other cultures through fieldwork in India, Thailand, and Costa Rica. I understand the power of culturally competent care in delivering sustainable and holistic treatments, and want to dedicate my life to empowering those in under-served areas.

Scientific Inquiry: I am in constant pursuit of learning and using the scientific process to integrate information. I am pursuing an honors thesis in nutrition to understand how we can improve health outcomes and reduce the burden of obesity in the US. I have honed my skills in the language of science to actively participate in scientific inquiry and discourse.

Ask Great Questions

The best way to interact with admissions officers, both in-person and online, is to ask good questions and really listen to the responses. These are questions that one would not normally find answers to on the school's website. It gets really tedious for admissions officers to answer questions that could easily be looked up. Your premed can distinguish herself by asking for real information that relates to her personal situation. Interesting questions can be about milestones in the application cycle that will be specific to that school (e.g. when are the last interview days?), initiatives that the representative is personally involved or invested in, and mentorship and student health at that school.

Current applicants can ask these good questions:

- When is your last interview day for this cycle?
- Are you still issuing interview invitations?
- As I am hoping to interview with you, and have done some research, service, clinical work, since I last connected with you, is it better to update you through email, through the AMCAS portal, or now through this chat?

Future applicants can ask these good questions:

- What innovations and changes in the student experience is your school anticipating over the next few years?
- How does faculty mentorship work at your school? Is it formal, as in students are assigned to mentors, or is it informal, and students find their own way to advisors and mentors?
- As an admissions officer, do you get to interact with the people you select as they go through their four years?
- If you had to choose one of these three as the most important primary selection factor for your school, which would it be: service, clinical experience, or research?
- Are you planning any open houses at the school this year?
- What fairs do you plan to attend in person?

- Could I arrange to visit you at the school sometime? (Only ask this if you actually think you might.)

Here are some not so interesting, more transactional questions for them to answer that might relate to your situation:

- What percentage (if any) of your class is selected through special programs, such as articulation agreements, early admissions programs or linkages with postbac programs?
- If the school is a state-funded institution: What percentage of the class are in-state residents?
- How do you view re-applicants reapplying in the next admissions cycle? And a follow-up: Do you offer post-cycle counseling for applicants who were not accepted?

You should definitely tailor these questions to your own situation, giving background and context before asking them.

Virtual Fairs

For networking in virtual spaces, professionalism in written communication is critical and it is important to have professional, friendly portraits to use online. Health Professions Week, held annually, is a good virtual place to learn directly what the schools are up to regarding their timing of interview invitations and where they will visit in person. The annual AAMC Virtual Medical School Fair is a big gift from the American Association of Medical Colleges (AAMC). Registration is free.

Many medical schools show up for pre-applicants, and applicants as well. For people who are early in the application cycle, or haven't applied yet, it is a place to find specific school information that will come in handy later when they are explaining why they are a good fit for a particular school in their essays. It is important to take note of information that may not be widely available or easily found on the schools' websites, including information about curricular reform, student initiatives, and culture. Your premed should choose their top 5 or 10 schools and think ahead of time of questions to ask them, as well as take down all the names and contact information they can get. Frequently, a medical school admissions officer will tell a pre-applicant to send an email to remind him that they met when she does submit an application to that school.

For people applying in the current application cycle, the medical school fair is designed as a place to connect meaningfully and personally with the admissions officers who will review their application. Applicants should connect with admissions officers at schools that they are still waiting to hear from. The probability may be low—but the possibility is real—that they could make a connection that leads to an interview. Applicants should use their real name when signing in and include their AAMC ID#, if they are a current applicant, in case the school representative wants to look up the applicant and offer an interview! Do not miss this opportunity! Nearly every year, several applicants I advise get a coveted interview invitation from meeting an admissions officer in virtual reality there.

Professional Online Presence

Here's an example of a 2018 tweet that popped up from someone I follow.

Twitter 10/28/18: C. Michael Gibson MD @CMichaelGibson "If you are a pre medical student, someone intending to pursue an MPH or PhD and would like to spend 2 or more years working with me in clinical trials please DM me."

A great job, advertised only on Twitter. Go and figure.

I was reluctantly pushed into the Twitter universe by Tom, an applicant-turned-medical student who had used it to great effect himself in maintaining a lucrative side hustle as a DJ through medical school and college. He told me that I usually ended an advising session with a pithy aphorism that he could take away and think about. He said these little Janet soundbites would make great tweets and I should spread the wealth. To be honest, I had not even been aware of my little tweetable closing remarks, and I resisted, saying they would be taken out of context. I also thought of Twitter as a coarse battleground megaphone for nasty people. Was I ever wrong.

Twitter is actually many things to many people, and the part of its universe that I now gladly inhabit is made up of people who want to share their intentions and happy news about making the world of medicine better for medical students, doctors and their patients. Most of the medical school admissions offices and certainly their public-facing news offices are all on Twitter. Many medical doctors use Twitter to express passing commentary on issues affecting healthcare today. The AAMC tweets to premeds and every other constituent body on a regular basis.

My own Twitter account is named @BigRedPremed, in honor of the school where I learned the most about premed advising, and because I like the rhyme-y sound of it. I only tweet about medical school admissions with the single exception that I retweet my daughter's tweets about her company, one which brings families into stronger community with each other and offers free tutoring to students who would otherwise lag behind. I don't tweet about the day I am having or other random observations. It's strictly a professional platform.

Every premed needs to launch a professional social media platform and Twitter is a great place to start. Social, or digital media, is a place to broadcast your career interests, and show your values, your character, and your thought leadership. You must separate your personal from your professional accounts. Many people use a slightly differently spelled surname on their personal accounts once they develop a professional presence. Executed correctly, presence on digital media shows a premed's professionalism, increases their visibility and credibility and gives people a chance to recognize their name when sifting through hundreds or even thousands of applications. A premed can use digital media to link together all the places that they have professional accounts on the internet, from LinkedIn to TikTok to Reddit. Use these accounts to follow people and organizations you admire, feel connected to, and want to connect with.

Conclusion

Networking gives other people a chance to care about your premed and their goals. They need to let them have their chance to help. People associated with the world of medicine want to see others succeed in a medical field so they in turn can help even more people. Before your premed knows it, they will be the one people are reaching out to for help. Your premed's chance to give back for all this help is right around the corner.

12 Crisis Management and Red Flags

It's no secret that a horrifyingly large percentage of students of all ages, from middle school to medical school, suffer from a disproportionate share of anxiety and depression. Student responses to campus social issues amidst the rigor of their schedule and activities drives up stressors and can precipitate serious meltdowns. Premeds don't get personal days. Mental health needs to be managed and addressed through many modalities. When an adverse campus event takes place, like a major sexual assault case or a suicide, students aspiring for health careers who are prone to anxiety and depression can be deeply triggered by these things. There can be personal situations, too, like a rejection, breakup or just a series of bad grades or even just a natural slump, that can trigger more serious mental conditions. Their best friend can become very needy and drain your own child's reservoir of wellness.

It is very important for parents to stay connected with their offspring, and to stay apprised of events on campus. Parents can read the student newspaper and join parent groups of college students so they know what's going on. Stay in touch with your child so you can develop a sense of when to intervene.

Medical schools want to know that any applicant who goes through those periods steadily gains tools they need to bring themselves back to balance and equanimity; that they work towards health and monitor themselves. The fact that a student experiences severe depression is not a reason to be rejected from school or hide the problem. What is important is that the student knows how the healing process works and that mental health is a lifelong challenge that will need to be continually addressed and managed.

Red Flags: Out, Out Damn Spot!

Medical schools require that people disclose a lot about themselves. I don't think there's a single person who is comfortable disclosing everything they have done in their lives, and there may be things your premed has been a part of or even instigated that you don't know about. Here are some ways to look at the stuff that's hard to share with a medical school admissions committee.

To you and your premed, a red flag is a blemish on their credentials. Like a pimple that shows up at an inopportune time, there may be a desire to attack the problem in ways that augment, rather than diminish it. Red flags need to be addressed with a cool head and a clear eye. To the medical school admissions committee, a red flag is a reason to pause and wonder if, despite all the great attributes and experiences in the application, maybe they would be better off going with the next person they review. The most common red flags include:

- An aberrant semester with either weak grades, withdrawals or incompletes
- Driving infractions, from rolling through a stop sign to driving under the influence
- Empty periods without "self development:" gaps in the academic record, summers not accounted for, or even periods of unaccounted for inactivity in the gap year after college

- Unprofessional behavior in a residential setting, like a dorm or apartment
- Unprofessional digital media presence, which could be on someone else's accounts (hacking)
- Personal oddities that may be noted in a letter of recommendation
- Poor judgment, noted in a letter
- Lack of integrity, noted in a letter or an institutional action record
- Actions that hurt someone else
- Breaking institutional rules, like burning candles in a residence hall

The primary application wording on the infractions question demands that even charges which were dropped or mistakenly leveled at your offspring should be reported.

The premed and their family are not the best to judge the seriousness of these red flags. Most likely, the premed will think it's much worse than it is, while the parent might want to reassure them that it is much less significant than it may be. Certainly, it's not the end of the world, but you don't know how significant it may prove to be. How can you tell then, what qualifies as an issue that rises to the level of damaging an application? Talk to a qualified person. The most important qualifications are:

- You have good reason to trust them
- Admissions committees have no relationship to them
- They know something about how admissions committees at different schools weigh and discuss these factors

How are red flags weighed in the admissions process and when do they come up? Red flags can enter the application process in several different ways. Some of these ways are within the premed's control and some are not. For those areas of the application that are in their control—disclosing it in their essays, interviews, and letters of recommendation—they can take a cautious approach, in consultation with an advisor, to framing the red flag. For parts of the application where one has less control over the content of the red flag—institutional records and background checks—the premed has to face that the situation will be viewed adversely and it may mandate a few more years before applying to put the incident behind them. It all depends on the people in the admissions office and how they view certain things, as well as who could have been hurt by the incident.

One medical school has a committee to assess just institutional actions. They have two guiding rules. 1) one infraction, we will talk it over; more than one similar infraction: rejection. 2) If the incident hurt the applicant, we will talk it over; if it could have hurt another person, even potentially: rejection.

Common issues are handled in routine ways. These include: Underage drinking on campus, grades below B in courses and other aberrant semester grades.

Uncommon issues are handled in sometimes unpredictable and hastily devised ways. These include more serious alcohol infractions, such as using a fake ID, or being even arrested and charged, much less convicted of a DUI and of course sexual harassment, assault and rape. Undergraduate chicanery is often weighed by looking at the campus judicial officer report, to see how the issue was weighed internally. Transgressions to characterize this way include stealing street signs, swimming in the off-limits and dangerous gorges at Cornell, scaling high campus towers on Halloween to mount pumpkins on spires, and non-alcohol hazing.

Academic integrity violations are taken very seriously and usually require the premed to wait a few years and engage in activities where they can show that they are honest people and have learned from their mistake. Integrity violations include cheating, forging letters of recommendations, and sadly, I have even seen transcript forging.

How to Frame a Red Flag

The way premeds write about their red flags depends to some degree on who else has recorded the situation, and where and how they described it. The worst advice about red flags ranges from these two poles: tell them everything, to the other: tell them nothing. I say this because when the premed reports every single detail, it's easy to sound like they are qualifying what they did wrong and/or making excuses for it. When they tell them nothing, they end up carrying a dark secret, which feels terrible, one that can be found out at the wrong time and really hurt their chances.

When the premed writes and speaks about red flags, they need to keep it simple, and say what they did, take responsibility and stay positive. The premed is almost never entirely to blame for the red flag, but when they implicate others and assign them blame, medical schools may see this as a lack of responsibility and maturity. The admissions committees, if they are willing to forgive the applicant for what they did in the first place, want to hear about a growth phase after the incident and the ability to talk about what they learned.

One of the worst red flags in academic integrity, one I have seen all too often, is when a frightened premed takes responsibility for something they actually did not do, because for one reason or another they felt intimidated at the time, or because they were aware of what was happening and feel really guilty that they did not stop it. I have seen people whose work others copied and turned in. They did not know about it until they were called up by the professor for turning in identical work. I have seen a kind premed share a homework assignment with a friend after his mother died suddenly and he had to leave campus, only to get called up on charges. I have seen freshman who innocently collaborated on a group project over video platforms during the pandemic only to be told by their professor that the extent of their collaboration went over the line.

And I have seen many, many students cheat, and get caught, only to have the professor dismiss the evidence because he did not want to take the time to deal with it. And I have heard over and over and over from premeds that they have seen others cheat in networks and not get caught.

There are so many nuances that we need to really understand what happened before we respond. Doctors need to be ethical people, and at the same time, we all make mistakes. All red flags are just character development waiting to happen. Your premed needs to be urged to turn his red flag into evidence of his resilience, to articulate what he learned from the situation in a heartfelt and candid manner.

One way to think of it: Turn your pain into your passion that is your purpose.

I was stressed out and overwhelmed. My newest friend invited me to try bourbon in his room. It was my first month of college. We were caught by the resident assistant and ultimately convicted of alcohol violations. During the mandated alcohol abuse training my school gave me as a sanction for my behavior, I learned why schools need to monitor underage drinking in their residence halls. They are actually protecting their students. I founded a club of volunteers, now funded by our university health services, students who attend off-campus parties as sober monitors, and warn the organizers of alcohol use and abuse so they can monitor their own parties and protect their guests.

Red Flags During the Application Process

You are implicated in something you have nothing to do with that takes time to be resolved…

You get pulled over speeding for a good reason…

You turn 21 and there's a party…

You are interviewing every week during your fall senior year semester and your grades tank…

Of all these, your premed needs to talk over the incident in detail with an advisor, who can help them understand and articulate its critical features. In general, as long as there is not a criminal record on background check, applicants have more latitude about how and when to inform the schools. If an applicant is worried about that, they can do their own background check to see if it's there and what it says. Gather all information before worrying and again, talk to an advisor who knows the medical school admissions process.

Successful Handling of Red Flags

The ten undergraduate transcripts, three with Ws (post deadline course withdrawals) all over them: Mary was a Division I athlete on scholarship, captain of her team, whose coach literally would not permit her to take the chemistry and physics courses that were offered during the season her sport competed. After she graduated, her college sweetheart was drafted into a professional sports league. He changed teams each year for three years and she took courses wherever she could find them. Once she registered in two places at two schools in different parts of the country, until they settled down. The medical schools were fine with her explanation.

The machete in the backpack on the Arts Quad: Topher was an avid wilderness guide. After leading a particularly exhausting trip, he went back to campus, went to class, then went outside and fell asleep in the grass. While he was asleep, his backpack was stolen. He reported it and when the campus police found it, without his money or his laptop, it had the machete he had used on his camping trip. He was reported for bringing a concealed weapon on campus. It took a long time to resolve and he explained it precisely on his applications. He had 14 interviews and got into his first choice school.

The incredible disappearing/reappearing academic integrity violation: Amanda was accused as a freshman, along with three other freshman women, of violating the code of academic integrity, by collaborating to a degree greater than permitted on a group project. She tried to plead her innocence and ignorance, but the faculty member convicted all four women and informed them in writing that the infraction would be noted on their permanent academic transcript. After that semester, the faculty member took a job at a different school. Amanda was never sure of whether to inquire about what happened next. She was worried that if she asked her institutional prehealth advisor about it, maybe gears that had ground to a halt would start up again.

Finally, she decided to order a transcript in her junior year as she considered whether to apply as a junior or senior to medical school. There was no mention on the transcript. Relieved, she decided to apply the following year, her senior year. She had a transcript ordered to give me because she had decided to work with me. The academic integrity violation was at that point on the transcript, to her horror. I learned that the registrar who first received the conviction from the departing faculty member had done nothing with it because it was not finalized until a committee authorized the action. Then that registrar left the school and a new registrar came in briefly, discovered the record, and put it on Amanda's transcript.

We decided that she would write to the committee that never formerly authorized the transcript notation and ask them to remove it on several grounds we noted. They agreed she had suffered enough, the record was expunged, Amanda applied to medical school and was accepted exactly where she wanted to go.

I could go on, but I will spare you. Stuff happens in institutions and often a strategic mind is required to organize an effective response. I don't suggest you hire a lawyer or try to work out something like this yourself. Leave it to someone you trust who understands these systems well

13 Assessing Timing, Readiness and Motivation

Live your life with gratitude for the past,
infinite attention to the present,
and responsibility for the future.

Families often feel itchy about when their premed should apply to medical school. Is it this summer? Is there a way that it can be this summer? If not this summer, will they lose their edge/interest/ability/motivation and never go to medical school? Let's examine this thought, from the point of view of reality. We have a path, which has already taken place, and may include some potholes and missed signals. We have a present moment, which may include distractions like family troubles, illness, significant others and their family troubles, illnesses or need for attention. We have a plan for the future. Try to keep the elements separate in considering the crucial decision to apply now or not. The path is not the plan. Let's not argue with reality; let's look right at it.

Bare Minimum Credentials

Your premed is ready to apply with some hope of acceptance to a medical school when all the following essential and minimum elements are in place:

- 75% of the premed prerequisite coursework is completed, as well as a plan for completing all within one year is in place. No grade can be below a C in these courses, and all grades must average at least a 3.0. Note that grades of C- and below generally do not fulfill medical school prerequisite requirements. If your child has such grades, he or she will need to retake the courses while, or better, before applying.
- An MCAT score result received by August 31 of the application year, that exceeds the 75th percentile for that application year. You can look up current percentiles on the AAMC website. Use the keywords "AAMC MCAT percentiles."
- A BCPM (Biology, Chemistry, Physics and Math) GPA above 3.0
- An AO (All other) GPA above 3.0
- A minimum of 2 medically oriented service experiences lasting more than 2 weeks that took place during the college years or later.
- A minimum of 2 non-medically oriented service experiences lasting more than 3 weeks that took place during the college years or later.
- Three letters of recommendation completed by July 1 of the application year from institutionally-situated faculty or staff, and former employment, internship, or volunteer supervisors. Usually one of these must be from someone who taught science to your premed.
- The applicant's schedule must contain at least three hours per day, or 18 hours per week, for application drafting and review, from May through July of the cycle.
- $1,250 must be available in capital or credit to pay for the primary and secondary application. Interviews at schools drive this much higher. Scholarships are available for families who can't afford these fees. If your family is in this situation, the best approach is to contact the medical school directly to learn how to get fees waived.

Essential Minimum Credentials

Most applicants who possess only these minimum credentials will not gain admission to medical school. Without possessing all of them, they are nearly guaranteed not to gain admission. To improve the chances to over 50%, the essential minimum elements look like this:

- 75% of the premed prerequisite coursework completed with no grade at or below a B and all grades averaging at least a 3.5, as well as a plan in place for completing all within one year. No more than two grades can be below a B (C+ or C only; no C-) in these courses, and all grades must average at least a 3.5.
- An MCAT score result received by July 15 of the application year that exceeds the 85th percentile for that application year.
- An AAMC-calculated BCPM (Biology, Chemistry, Physics & Math) GPA above 3.4
- An AAMC-calculated AO (all other) GPA above 3.2
- A minimum of two medically oriented service experiences lasting more than 3 weeks that took place during the college years or beyond.
- A minimum of two non-medically oriented service experiences lasting more than 3 weeks that took place during the college years or beyond.
- Three letters of recommendation completed by July 1 of the application year from institutionally-situated faculty or staff, and former employment, internship, or volunteer supervisors. Usually one of these must be from someone who taught science to your premed.
- The applicant's schedule must contain at least three hours per day for application drafting and review, or a minimum of 18 hours per week from May through July of the cycle.

- $5000 in available credit or cash for the primary application, secondary fees and any in-person interview.

To further improve the chances, just increase the amounts in each item on the list. What if your premed does not have these elements? The simplest way to improve one's chances in the face of insufficiency is to take advantage of the thing you can control: give the premed more time. Take another year or two, go through the list and make a plan for strengthening the areas that fall below the recommended levels.

In other words, don't frame this application process as "now or never," not on any level in your own heart and mind. The time to apply is either now or later. Your premed deserves the chance to honestly evaluate their admissions chances with your support.

Be forewarned that the decision to apply now or to extend the plan for another year or two contains some subterranean power politics. Aside from your own expectations and that of other important people in your premed's life, aside from how they filters and uses those expectations to fuel their own motivations–or resistance–other people loom over the decision.

The Prehealth Advisor's Opinion

Your premed ought to ask the college premed advisor for an opinion on her readiness. She should schedule the conversation at the start of the academic term that just precedes the summer when she hopes to apply, thus giving her a few months to enact the standard or revised plan. The college premed advisor may have an opinion, which is well worth seeking. You can gain a sense of the advisors' expertise on readiness by suggesting that your premed ask her advisor about the outlier successes. "Can you tell me about some students who successfully gained admission when their numbers did not predict success? What factors helped them?"

Whatever opinion the advisor gives your premed, green light, yellow light or red light, don't let your premed walk away feeling like the advisor said she's not medical school "material." Don't blame the advisor if your premed feels this way after the talk. It might be a miscommunication: Ultimately your premed's feelings after the advising talk reveal a confidence issue. Sooner or later, your premed is going to have to develop such unshakable inner confidence in the plan that nobody can even give her a whiff of the impression that she's "not medical school material."

The advisor can only provide an opinion based on their information, knowledge, curiosity and concern for your premed. If any of these areas are lacking, it's probably not the advisor's fault. It's just too bad. Premed advising is an intense business, and nearly all premed advisors are seriously overworked and under-supported themselves. Give the advisor credit for what is offered. Just remember that whatever the advisor decrees about your premed's readiness, it is nobody's business but the medical school admissions office to offer the seat or deny the seat.

Asking Family Friends and Connections

You may have a family friend whom you think knows something because of a connection. If you are lucky, this appointed premed guide will have a sense of what they know and do not know, how far their influence extends, and the limits of their reach in this regard. Unfortunately, many do not. Even doctors who sit on admissions committees have a painfully limited view of the whole selection process. Depending on their relationship with you, and their own need to be needed and helpful, they can really derail your true perspective. They can completely undermine a knowledgeable institutional advisor's wisdom. They can intrude and intervene in ways that are at best embarrassing and at worst can derail admissions chances at a school for your premed. Be really careful about bringing them into the potpourri.

When it comes to family friends and connections, it is for you to do the calling and talking. You vet that person's value to your child. Do not depend on these ad hoc advisors for the now or later consideration. They don't know the factors that weigh into readiness and, further, they cannot take the care with this decision that your premed and you will. Nearly all the time, these family network connections will help you to become a wiser guide. Don't demand that your child meet with them. Only make connections when you are absolutely sure that your premed will gain confidence from meeting these people in your network.

Responding to Emotional Fallout of a Readiness Conversation

It is unprofessional for an advisor to tell an applicant that he or she will never gain admission to medical school. In fact, don't even believe your premed if he says this is what he heard. The advisor needs to be honest, and thus might give the impression that your premed, in his opinion, is not yet suitable for medical school. It's very, very hard and out of character for a helping professional to actually state those cruel and devastating words. It is far more likely that your premed went in fearing that he would hear this and looked for confirmation. If he said he did hear this, don't belabor it.

Instead, give this message: *It must have been devastating to hear that. Is it true? Is the advisor a medical school admissions officer? I don't believe that you can't get into a medical school. I believe that you can. I suggest that you not believe it either. Why don't you tell me what part of that prophecy you do believe so we can modify the plan to eradicate that possibility?*

Rigorously avoid criticizing the messenger: *The advisor is not worth listening to. The advisor is bad. The advisor is not knowledgeable. The advisor does not care about you.*

You think you are providing unconditional love and acceptance by being on your premed's side, but you may actually be contributing to the crisis of confidence triggered by the meeting with the advisor. When a confidence crisis arises, ask questions to get at whether they really believe it is true that they have no chance of achieving their cherished dreams. Make sure that they know that for as long as they want it, you believe in them. You believe in your premed; together you will take responsibility for the future. Embedded in that is your unconditional love and acceptance, not only of them, but of their dreams, from which they have fashioned their identities in the present.

The "red light: do not apply now" opinion on the part of an advisor is often based mostly on the extent to which the advisor knows your premed and their path to medical school. This is another in a host of reason why premeds need to proactively build meaningful relationships with advisors, even if the chemistry does not feel so great as they get "shuffled in and shuffled out" of their fifteen-minute advising appointments and generic info sessions, as my advisee, Penny, now a physician, so memorably put it. It is also based on at least some of the institutional elements imposed by the culture of the advisor's employer, *aka* the institution to which you are paying those many thousands of dollars of tuition, room and board. Even if the advisor is not that great at assessing your premed's readiness, they can still be phenomenally great at any number of other elements of successfully advising premeds, so don't write them off.

Ready or Not?

This is one of the most important questions in the application process. Pushing and trying just for the luck of it is a bad move. When your premed applies, they will take great personal pride in the outcome, and spend a lot of time and money. If nobody accepts them after all that, it can feel devastating. In addition, medical schools don't really want to see an application year after year. If they reject an applicant, they expect them to spend a year strengthening their application. The decision to apply before one is ready can and frequently does result in needing to wait until way after one is ready, because of this. The readiness decision is a family decision, with the premed holding the tie-breaking vote. It is their life after all. What we hope is that the premed will have the wisdom and discernment to apply in the one cycle when their chances of success are greatest.

14 Taking More Time: A Gap Year, Bridge Year, Launch Year

As I described in an earlier chapter, I recommend that applicants at the outset consider the scenario where they take one year before applying to medical school, thus two gap years before entering medical school. In addition to the opportunity for the applicant to become even better prepared to succeed in the application cycle, many familial and personal health reasons may influence one to take gap years. So, what is a premed to do between college and medical school? It should definitely be something, and likely one of the activities below, because they will want to explain the gap between graduation and matriculation in their application, and they should have a good story of personal growth and service to show for that time.

Academic Enhancement

Academic enhancement after college should only be contemplated if your premed's academic record is less than stellar and the student is highly motivated to improve it. Some students will have received poor grades because they didn't apply themselves, so their only real option is to attend medical school in the Caribbean (but be advised that this path in some respects just pushes out farther the challenge of becoming a physician, because they'll have to become very high achieving at their

Caribbean school to have a chance at residency in the US). Another reason for academic enhancement after college is that the applicant is missing critical prerequisite courses. And another reason is if the most recent grades are not mostly As (75%) or there are Cs in junior or senior year (organic chemistry is the exception). A weak ending of college is highly problematic, whereas an upward trend in grades from freshman to senior year is acceptable.

Many programs are eager to take your 50k to rehabilitate your premed's academic record. But you must be careful about choosing the right program, because not all academic enhancement post-baccalaureate (a program completed after graduation from college) programs will serve as a vehicle to get your premed to medical school. They vary tremendously in quality and price. Many of them, in order to close the deal, advertise incentives such as the so-called articulation agreements with medical schools (an agreement that the medical school will give the postbac student a guaranteed interview—sometimes even a guaranteed seat), which may or may not be active options at the time your premed tries to exercise them.

So how do you find a good postbac program? This is really an area where a knowledgeable advisor can help guide you to the right programs. But if you don't have access to someone like that, in general, the best programs have their own prehealth and career advisors who will speak to you and your premed before you apply. I always recommend the Temple University College of Science and Technology (CST) Postbac Program and suggest you look at it first, to learn what a truly well-structured program with outstanding advising offers its students. Temple has a few programs; make sure you search for the CST one. Founded by Grace Hershman, an icon in the prehealth advising world, an advisor to the advisors, you can compare all others to the dream program that she developed there. It is important that your premed speaks with the advisor at the school they select. They need to feel that they can relate really well to the advisor because they will be working closely together. If an advisor doesn't have time to talk to the premed before they apply, it's probably not a program they can feel certain is right for them.

Some programs are one year long, others are two years long. However many years they last, it's important to consider that it may be better to wait a year after finishing the postbac to apply to medical school. The reason not to apply directly upon graduating is that most postbac programs don't end in time for the applicant to be ready to apply in May. Additionally, many programs encourage students to take the MCAT in the summer after the postbac program is finished, which then delays their application to medical school. If a student is trying to complete their postbac and prepare for the MCAT and write their medical school application, they could once again hit the same traffic jam that caused them to get poor grades in the first place. Plan out the postbac and application cycle timeline with your premed ahead of time.

There are several things to watch out for when evaluating postbac programs. Some programs seem to be a way for a school to bring in a ton of revenue without having to matriculate a student with the same resource demands as a normal undergraduate. In this case, the postbac student may feel like a second class student, lacking access to services at the school like the fitness center, counselling, or health clinic. This is something to check out in advance because it's certainly not stated up front.

The other thing to find out is whether the program has stand-alone courses or if postbac students take the same courses as undergraduates. It would not be very helpful to take another 300-student biology course with competitive premeds, if the goal is to get a good grade in the course, when your student could be in a postbac course with 30 students who are all in the same boat. Not to mention, a postbac student may be in the situation of competing with undergraduate students to even enroll in the course, and it would be devastating to be shut out of a needed course. Another thing to watch out for is how individualized the program is so that your premed doesn't have to retake classes where they already achieved a good grade.

Other postbac programs, in their well-intentioned attempt to make a program that will definitely get the premed into a better position to apply, offer the chance to take classes like physiology alongside medical students. While the idea is to prove that your student can achieve in medical school because they have already taken medical school courses with med students, the problem is that medical students are more qualified than your premed and have a higher incentive to do better. Therefore, the competition, like in college, makes it unnecessarily challenging for your premed to get good grades (which is the whole point of doing this). You can learn material and get good grades without subjecting yourself to competition with a cohort of people who are far more experienced at doing that than you are. Relative grading is not representative of mastery, but both grades and mastery are what we are looking for, so take classes at an institution where you can actually get good grades.

Career Changers

The career changer postbac programs are for students who studied something completely outside of science and have not taken more than a couple of the premed prerequisites in college, students who studied such subjects as English, Theater, Fine Arts, Engineering and anyone else who has had an epiphany that it is their calling to become a physician. These programs will provide all the science prerequisites. Another type of student is a premed attending a large college who decides that they don't want to take premed courses there because the class sizes are so large and graded on a mean. They don't want to compete in that way. So students can major in something else and then do a career changer postbac program.

Career changer programs are very selective, so they generally have a cohort of talented, smart and dedicated students. Students in these programs have to study constantly and essentially do not have time for anything else. If your premed enrolls in a career changer program, they should take a year off afterwards to study for the MCAT and engage in clinical experiences. Don't be seduced at the outset by the thought that after that first year you can apply to medical school; this route really takes three years to be successful unless you are selected for a very competitive articulation agreement match. These are a few spots that the program has negotiated that make it easier to apply for and gain admission to a few select schools. As mentioned earlier, please be wary of this offer as they may not be active options at the time your premed wants to use them.

Special Master's Programs

As a way to rehabilitate grades, Special Master's Programs (SMPs) are designed to help prehealth students, not just premeds, to enhance their academic record. The best programs for a premed help develop the student's medical school narrative in other areas, too, through opportunities to conduct research or earn an EMT certification to show in-depth clinical exposure. Research-oriented SMPs are often designed to populate research labs on campus with extremely hard-working, motivated premeds. What then may happen is that a task-master researcher demands that your student spend long hours in the lab (because things rarely go according to plan when you are conducting research) when your premed should be studying for exams. Since the strategic objective of taking the program is to get good grades in courses, sometimes the demands of research scientists on their lab assistants can cause students in this program to experience a lot of task friction—and threaten to defeat the primary purpose of taking the program in the first place, which was to enhance the student's GPA.

Also, sometimes research programs require a thesis—and while this might sound like a shiny object to flash on a medical school application, the thesis is not usually finished at the time of submitting the primary application. Sometimes the thesis is held up by lab work the student still needs to accomplish (because things are not going according to plan, as mentioned above) and the project extends through summer, through the start of the application cycle, and your student does not have time to get their application to medical school submitted on time. Research is not a critical requirement for medical school, but it is great to have, so be cautious about these programs.

SMPs have a critical distinction from postbac programs. While grades earned in the postbac program will be considered as part of the undergraduate grade point average, grades derived during an SMP will be listed as a separate line on the medical school application, as a graduate GPA. This matters because if a student's undergraduate GPA is below ~3.2, it will be almost impossible for a one or two year postbac to rehabilitate their GPA to the point that an algorithm that screens GPAs on medical school applications will take note of their achievement.

The academic record from an SMP or other graduate program is a standalone line on the medical school application that will show exactly how well the student did. That applicant's accomplishment will be obvious, the medical school algorithm will be stumped, and this will force the admissions office to review the application manually. Thus, if the applicant's cumulative science GPA is below ~3.2, and does not trend straight upwards after a weak beginning, an SMP is probably a preferable route to medical school admissions.

Other Ways to Enhance an Academic Record

I sometimes recommend that an applicant design a DIY (do-it-yourself) postbac program to enhance an undergraduate GPA by enrolling in undergraduate courses. They can matriculate at the least expensive nearby state school. They can go to many schools at once. The student will simply take courses that they need to retake or those additional ones they need to enhance their record. They can even take online courses, although they shouldn't do them all online. With the DIY method, you can pay by the course. Naturally, as an advisor, I recommend that you secure good advising. You can ask your former institutional advisor if they will continue to work with you, or find an independent advisor to help you with your course selection and explain how to secure the recommendations and complete the requirements that you need to be a successful medical school applicant.

The second type of DIY postbac is to apply to an undergraduate school to obtain a second bachelor's degree (BA/BS). Even though your premed already has an undergraduate degree, many schools will allow them to transfer in the courses that they used to earn that degree and allow them to become an undergraduate there. They have so-called residency requirements to earn the second degree which range from one to two years of full-time study. When your premed becomes an undergraduate there, they will qualify for financial aid and become a first class undergraduate citizen at that school, first in line to get the courses they need. Your premed will also benefit from their academic and prehealth advising, which is great. And they can get a whole additional degree.

Your premed also doesn't have to satisfy all the school's degree requirements, then graduate and receive a second B.A. What matters to the medical schools is that they took several courses each semester and got mostly As. The applicant already has a degree from the first school, and they can leave before the second bachelor's degree is complete with their academic transcript intact. It's a great method.

Research

If your premed does not need to enhance their record, but they would like to do research and build a great professional network before attending medical school, the NIH Intramural Research Program is an excellent opportunity. In this program, students apply to enter a lab at the NIH that interests them and do research (usually for two years). This program has an office of academic advising for people who plan to get medical degrees or PhD's in science that offers great programming all year long to provide community and opportunities for applicants as they prepare for medical school. The research experience is outstanding and the researchers tend to understand that applicants are applying to medical school and don't force them to overwork during their application year.

There are many standalone (no coursework) research opportunities for graduates who are preparing to apply to medical school. Labs are aware that they can recruit outstanding research assistants who want to take a year off to enrich their credentials for application to medical school. These research jobs consist of a wide range of activities and skills. The very best research position, in my view, is the job of clinical research coordinator. As a clinical research coordinator, the premed not only learns about research as it relates directly to improving medical care, they also get to meet patients and develop their communication skills, which is of critical importance to medical school admissions. A research coordinator recruits and educates patients, consents them for the research project, and follows up with them over time to ensure they are following the protocols of the research study. Thus, premeds who take these positions get a lot of clinical science experience.

They also get a fair amount of experience working with the people who support the scientists who administer these studies, and develop interprofessional skills. Often, medical schools are concerned that aspiring doctors only want to hang out with, or only respect other doctors. In this type of role, your premed can demonstrate that they have cooperated with a wide range of professionals all working together to take care of patients and complete the study. Clinical research coordinators often work in hospitals, which gives them tremendous access to other clinical settings and to network with physicians and hospital administrators. It is a great place to meet other physicians and ask for the opportunity to observe procedures and clinical rounds, as well as parts of hospital life that would be closed off otherwise, if they were not an insider at the hospital due to their job.

The way to find a clinical research coordinator role is to check out websites of large centers of medical education and teaching hospitals. Many of these positions are actually located at medical schools, so your premed will naturally have proximity to people who know the people in the medical school admissions committee.

Scribes and Other Direct Clinical Work

Premeds who need to spend dedicated time increasing their exposure to clinical medicine can seek work as a scribe, medical assistant or doctor's assistant. Physicians love hiring premeds in their gap years as clinical assistants because they are excellent employees and it brings them back to fond memories of their own training and the mentorship they found there. It's pretty easy to get these jobs, and because they vary in suitability and culture, the premed should look around at many before choosing one. The pay is low, but the future value is high. You can find hiring agencies that do scribe placement on the internet. Dermatologists particularly like to hire scribes because their medical specialty licenses allow them to train their assistants to do more clinical procedures than most medical assistants are permitted within their range of practice. The premeds like this work, too! Nothing more fun than draining an abscess or freezing off a skin tag! Sometimes physicians advertise on large employment message boards like Indeed or Craigslist.

Interest-Based Activities

Interest-based activities are anything that has been an abiding interest of your premed for some time that they would like to pursue full-time or half-time between college and medical school. Some of these activities may include getting a master's degree in music performance, joining the Peace Corps, or traveling to another country and engaging in service there. Your premed could decide to teach and mentor others as an athletics coach at their high school or college alma mater, or join Teach for America or Americorps to teach in inner city schools. City Corps, Americorps, City Year and the Medical Reserve Corps all provide paid opportunities for premeds to make a difference, gain proximity to human suffering, and learn the means for alleviating it on micro and macro levels.

One of my favorite sites for finding engaging work in social justice combined with interests in subjects such as fine art, building construction, and nutrition is Idealist.org. It lists volunteer and paid opportunities for differing levels of experience and training.

Gap years are a great time for a student to invest in themselves, grow as a person, save money, help others, and spend time with their family and friends before medical school. The only thing that medical schools don't like about a year spent between graduating and matriculating is time spent doing nothing. If that year is spent working for a community agency, great. If your premed cared for a sick or aging family member, that is a legitimate way to spend their time. The most important thing is to do something that can be documented and supports your premed's narrative as a caring person and excellent clinical communicator who is ready to become a doctor.

Medical schools appreciate applicants who step out of school for awhile. For parents, this is often a difficult prospect to entertain. Medical schools like students who have lived as autonomous professional adults, managing budgets and cooking for themselves, and had a chance to show how they would like to spend their time without the structure of school. There will be no stain whatsoever on the applicant who does this. In fact, it is most often seen as a sign of mental wellness and good judgment. I would like to close by sharing this first-person statement sent to me by my applicant, now Dr. Anat Chemerinski, to share with others debating the gap year decision, because it was Anat who convinced me that gap years are great:

GAP YEAR = BEST DECISION EVER

> *By freshman year, I was fairly certain about applying to medical school, so I couldn't think of any reason to take a gap year. While the Peace Corps, Teach for America, research and all of the other gap year possibilities sounded exciting, med school did too, and I wanted to get there as soon as possible. But during my sophomore and junior years, I realized I just didn't have enough time: time to study calmly for the MCAT, time to space out the premed requirements so that I could do as well as possible in those difficult classes, time to complete the primary application, the secondary applications, time to fly around for interviews. I also realized that after only three years in college, my application was not, realistically, as strong as it needed to be in this very competitive process.*

I had done a bit of research at Cornell and over the summer, but I knew research to be one area of my application that needed serious beefing up.[17] *I also realized that the contribution of my senior year science GPA would help me to be a more competitive applicant, and that I needed time to get my MCAT scores back. The more I thought about it, the more I saw holes in my application that could be patched during a gap year. I applied for a position as a research fellow at the NIH and I planned to volunteer at a hospital and to shadow an orthopedist as a way to get more clinical exposure. Basically, although I knew I wanted to go to medical school, I wanted to make sure the schools could see through my classes, activities, and experiences that I had really thought about what I was getting myself into.*

The medical school application process is long. Very long. It starts about a year and a half or two years before you actually matriculate. It's a huge commitment, and it involves enormous expenditures of time, energy, and money. It's stressful and disheartening at times, and wonderfully rewarding at others. It's not something to jump into before you are ready. For some people, a gap year is an opportunity to decide whether to apply to medical school, graduate school, neither, or both. For others, it's an opportunity to strengthen their application. It can also be a fantastic way to recover from the demanding Cornell premed coursework (mental health is important too!).

I'm having a most amazing gap year. I work from 8-4 and have all afternoon free to go out to dinner, see my friends, read, watch TV. I have time to exercise and sleep. I have time to enjoy traveling for interviews, and I know that I am more relaxed and focused during the interviews because I have nothing else to worry about. I would fully recommend taking a gap year to everyone.

---

17 This is only the case when one wants to attend a research-heavy school, or to become a physician scientist.

Many people go straight into medical school without a problem and are very happy with the decision. But it shouldn't be the default choice. Evaluate yourself as an applicant. Be honest with yourself and realistic about your position. Ask yourself: How do I know I want to go to med school? What concrete steps have I taken to figure this out? Have I had exposure to the medical profession? Have I had experiences that reflect my interest in the field? Will medical schools see all of this in my application? Or are there areas that could be improved? Research? Clinical exposure? Leadership? Volunteer work?

Perhaps you've been able to ask and answer these questions during your time at Cornell, and are ready to apply during your senior year. But if you haven't, consider taking a gap year. It will give you time to strengthen your application, to explore medicine- and non-medicine-related activities, to determine whether you are really ready for and interested in medical school, and it will give you time to watch The Office, guilt-free.

15 Overview of The Application Cycle

The application cycle is a long process that must be well-coordinated. There are times when nothing is happening and times when things move very fast, when it seems like everything cannot possibly get done.

Here is a list of what applicants should be thinking about and working on throughout the application cycle so you know what your premed will be going through. In general, applications for allopathic and osteopathic medical schools follow the same schedule with a few deviations that you can determine by looking at the important application dates published on the application service website, and at the deadlines for specific schools. For a planful premed, the application cycle begins in the fall before the summer that your applicant intends to submit their application.

Here is the timetable your premed should follow:

November

Schedule and prepare for the MCAT, which should be taken no later than next June, but January is far better.

Make a written plan, with contingencies for alternate approaches, to address any remaining weak areas in the candidacy over the next year. Work on committee letter materials if the school writes a committee letter.

Develop the narrative (we will discuss how to do this in a later chapter).

Prepare supplemental materials (resume, list of competencies the writer can attest to and how the applicant developed these) to give to the people whom they will be asking for letters of recommendation (LoR).

Attend networking events, info sessions, and fairs, and start building connections with students, staff, and faculty.

Journal regularly about experiences and ideas.

December

Study for the MCAT.

Ask mentors and professors if they will write a letter and give them the prepared supplemental materials. Consider when faculty get busy and don't give them a deadline that coincides with this. The deadline can be set any time through May, letters need to be finished by June.)

January

Read through the applicant guide or manual on how to fill out the application—it will be available online (AMCAS, AACOMAS, or TMDSAS).

Start writing the personal statement and activity descriptions for the application.

Make a digital media branding plan for the application cycle and beyond. Get on Twitter! Follow all the medical schools! See what's going on in the virtual medical education community!

February

Subscribe to MSAR (MD only) to begin research for choosing which medical schools to apply to. Look at the free medical school database at the Savvy Premed website.

Attend Health Professions Fairs. Check the calendar for leads at premedadvisor.com, and please, dear Reader, send us any you find that are not listed there!

March

Finalize the personal statement.

Pre-write secondaries for top ten schools.

April

Plan or start new activities to include in update letters that will be sent in the fall after applications are submitted.

Collect official transcripts from ALL schools attended to double check academic record and understand how long the transcript request process takes.

Confirm deadlines for submitting the primary application and individual schools.

May

Initiate primary application and begin to fill it in.

Send official transcripts to the primary application service.

Continue to pre-write secondaries.

Prepare for and reserve CASPer test if required by schools on the school list.

Submit primary application on the first day!

June

Ensure that LoRs are uploaded to the primary application.

Finalize the school list in the primary application.

Finalize secondary essay drafts.

July

Receive and submit secondary applications within two weeks of receiving them.

Read and listen to podcasts about medical ethics and current issues in medicine to prepare for interview questions.

Start or work in earnest on a capstone project for update purposes.

Keep journaling about experiences to use during interviews.

August

Continue submitting secondaries.

Check application status at schools applied to.

September

Prepare for and attend interviews through March.

Start new activities, excel at ongoing ones, and prepare a strategy to send update letters to schools.

Check online for nearby or virtual info sessions and fairs.

October

Medical schools begin to make application decisions (interview, hold, admit, waitlist, reject).

November

Send update letters to schools.

Attend health professions fairs to make connections with admissions officers and ask for an interview.

December

Be prepared for things to get very quiet the last three weeks of this month if you are in the application cycle.

January

Create a strategy for remainder of application cycle (withdraw, update, commit to enroll)

Family and applicant submit tax returns early.

Check with schools about financial aid applications.

February and March

Interviews come to a close in general; update to get off waitlists.

April and May

Admitted applicants notify schools of their decision by the deadline and withdraw from other schools.

Applicants on waitlists begin to be notified of changes in status: admissions offers and rejections.

Applicants who did not get accepted need to decide if they have improved their application enough over the last year that they are ready to apply again.

August

School orientation and the school year begins.

Timing of the Primary Application

In addition to the content of the primary application discussed in another chapter, the timing of submission is critical. The pressure to submit the primary application to AMCAS on the very first day or soon thereafter is legitimate, yet it can feel burdensome and confusing. Like most aspects of medical school admissions, your applicant's best action depends on many factors. The two most important questions to ask first are:

1. Is the primary application well-written and complete? Quality is more important than timing, but if your applicant has planned well, these don't have to be in conflict. Medical schools know this.
2. What other factors might hold up the application and make it irrelevant that my applicant submit as early as possible? These include MCAT score release and transcript receipt dates.

While most advisors cite the rolling admissions policy at medical schools as the chief reason to submit as early as you can, this is not the only important reason to do so. Rolling admissions means that, as one dean memorably stated, "the last seat in the class is the hardest to get."

After the application is submitted, the application service will verify the applicant's grades by cross-referencing them with all of the transcripts they submitted. The AMCAS transcript verification queue is dependent on the date of submission and receipt of transcripts, which the applicant should plan to arrive at the application service prior to hitting "Submit" on their application. Verification lag time naturally gets extended as the season progresses. I have been to AAMC and seen how they manually verify transcripts. It is time consuming. You want to be in the front of that queue. If, after they begin verification, the service finds that your applicant has not submitted all of their transcripts from every school or program they attended that provides a transcript, the application will be sent to the back of the line, behind thousands of other applications.

The other relevant queue is the one at many undergraduate and postbac schools for writing committee letters for their applicants. Some schools queue up their letter writing based on AMCAS submission. An applicant's application will not be complete at medical schools until letters are received and transcripts are verified, and other elements are submitted that I cover below. The applicant will not begin receiving secondary applications until the primary application is complete.

Finally, many admissions officers and committees take the position that people who apply early are good time managers, which is a critical skill in medicine. It is well-documented that mistakes are more often made, and judgment is more often compromised, by medical students and physicians whose organizational skills are lagging. In fact, admissions officers will cite studies of the strong correlation between medical malpractice and weak time management skills. Sometimes an applicant's submission dates are aired at the committee level when deciding between candidates, as evidence that one is better organized than the other. It is important to know that the admissions committees differentiate elements of the application you can control, for which you can be held accountable, from those you cannot.

After the primary application is submitted, additional elements can hold up the review of the application. Chief among these is submission of the secondary application. Applicants can find archived secondary questions online to guide them in prewriting secondary responses, so they can be nearly ready to submit when the prompts are formally made available to them.

Additional Required Assessments

Another element of the complete application is the CASPer online situational judgment test, which was introduced into the admissions process in 2010 and is required by more schools each year. Applicants sign up for a seat, take the test, and three weeks later, the school receives their score. The AAMC has spent ten years in development of their own situational judgment test, which was used in the 2022 admissions cycle for the first time. Altus Assessments, which develops and administers CASPer, has also found some adoption traction of the two online tests in their "suite," Duet and Snapshot.

Snapshot is a virtual, video-recorded online interview that admissions officers can review on their own schedule. Duet is a test of school mission fit, which asks applicants to choose between two alternatives, often program elements, that matter to them as they envision their training. To give a gross example, a Duet item might ask a test taker to say which is more important in medical school, early clinical exposure or early research opportunities. These tests serve two purposes. They provide data for schools to rate their admissions selection process against future success in medical school at various touch points, such as staying in good standing, exam scores, and clinical rotation ratings.

Applying Early

Many routes to medical school remind me of iconic children's board games. Candyland, as well as Chutes and Ladders, subtly teach children that life is full of hurdles, but by luck they can find shortcuts to speed up their route to reach the goal of being the first to finish the game. I wonder if the four year old who finishes first ever regrets winning the game, because then it's all over and no game is left to play.[18] The shortened routes include these:

Early Assurance, offered to sophomore applicants at select schools with different rules and conditions. These give the sophomore a pretty secure guarantee of admission straight out of college, often allowing them to avoid the MCAT and the normal application cycle, in exchange for knowing where they will attend medical school. Early Assurance usually sounds binding but it isn't. In general, but not always, it is a way to recruit the strongest applicants to a school early and to gain their loyalty.

Early Decision is a program where applicants only apply to one school, complete the application and are notified of the binding decision earlier than most applicants. This is a binding decision and if accepted, the applicant cannot change their mind in that cycle and apply elsewhere. If they are deferred or rejected, they then face applying late in that cycle and being behind everyone else. Early Decision for that reason is a big risk at most schools that offer it. The Rutgers New Jersey Medical School runs a program that is not nearly so risky and accepts many applicants. They are a shining exception. The benefits of Early Decision are fewer costs for medical school applications and a greatly eased pathway to medical school.

---

18 I wonder if this feeling of emptiness at the end of the admissions cycle, after years of gearing up for it, helps to explain why so many young doctors offer guidance with medical school admissions as a side occupation. Did the game of getting in require so much learning from them that they now want to share it and earn a little for their hard work?

Most institutional prehealth advisors strongly and unilaterally warn students against applying in this way. I have seen many successfully gain admission through this system and some stunning disappointments. In my experience, the admissions officer will give the applicant interested in Early Decision a preview conversation to give them a sense of whether they will be successful. The applicant really needs to listen and pay attention to their guidance. If the premed advisor has cultivated a strong and trusting relationship with the admissions officer, they can also learn the likelihood of acceptance.

The traditional path to medical school is long and fraught with many challenges. Premeds need to plan and to execute that plan with few slip-ups or lapses. They often need to sacrifice summer vacations the year they apply, or spend those vacations glued to their laptops, hunting for a wifi signal while they dispatch their vacation mates to hunt for the best margaritas. Such is the life of the noble premed in their application year.

16 Building the Narrative

Every story reveals information about your view of the world, your choices, and your priorities. Stories bring your passions and beliefs to life by showing what you have done about them.

~Carol Barash (Write out Loud, 2013)

What is a narrative? It's the story of who your applicant really is––in admissions office language. It's the answer to beautiful questions about what drives her, sustains her and energizes her. What are some of these beautiful questions?

- How do you use the lessons of your mentors to guide your actions in the world?
- When did you first discover the joy of having a healing impact on someone else's life?
- Why does a career in medicine excite and energize you?

All of the introspection work in this chapter will come in handy later in the personal statement, secondary application essays, interview preparation, and staying in touch with medical schools after the application is done.

Authenticity and Confidence

Eleanor is the daughter of a doctor and a lawyer. She has always attended the best private schools in Boston and is now at Ivy U. Throughout her education, Mom watched her stumble and watched her thrive. When she stumbled, Mom brought in the troops: counselors, teachers, private tutors, educational psychologists, coaches, personal trainers, admissions consultants. Every gap was carefully closed, with lasting results. When Dad learned the college admissions game, he invited Eleanor to get involved in community service, interesting summer experiences, and advanced coursework. Since college, she has kept her finger on the pulse of medical school admissions, always plumping her resume with service trips, summer internships, research, student activities, leadership, and clinical exposure. She has done so much.

Her parents paved the way—and paid the way. All this has been fine, until now. She doesn't believe that she has truly earned those credentials and whenever she sits down to write, she feels like a fake. This inner sense of inauthenticity and lack of confidence are common among consciously privileged applicants.

Imogene has a perfect GPA from Ivy U. She is a tireless and prodigious learner, a curious science-lover, and a meticulous student. Imogene has volunteered at the local free clinic for four years and now has the senior volunteer position there, supervising other volunteers and helping the organization set their volunteering needs. Imogene is personable, well-organized and dependable. I would call her deeply committed, a natural leader, and a grounded human being. When Imogene starts her application, she will shun all those words because she doesn't want to boast.

As a parent, how do you redirect this inner critic so the premed can talk with depth and feeling about their experiences? You start with the insight that your premed may feel this way but not want to share it with you. That might seem to them to be ungrateful, even disrespectful. Second, the job now is to usher one's self from what many call the "doing" mode to the "being" mode.

Everything your child did was done for reasons. The superficial reasons may have been to get into medical school, but all of them were choices. Some activities they really enjoyed, some they may have felt drained by, and they need to understand why in both cases.

Medical School Narrative

Medical school admissions officers want to understand each applicant's journey to a career in medicine, and how each event, activity, and idea leads to the next—this is called the narrative. Your child will share her narrative with admissions officers through the activities list, essays, and interviews. When we mention the process of "building the narrative," we are referring to the process your premed must go through to learn how to tell the story of how her personal qualities, background, and chosen activities have shaped who she is as a person who is ready to apply for medical school.

These are qualities that admissions officers look for in their applicants, and the parts of your premed's story that this chapter seeks to identify:

- Her goals and interests
- The ways she has demonstrated personal initiative through leadership, creativity, research, community service, motivation, or other life experiences
- The ways she has demonstrated motivation for and understanding of a career in medicine through academic achievement, exposure to clinical medicine, and community service
- The ways she has demonstrated good judgment, compassion, selflessness, and caring for others through extracurricular activities, personal and professional interactions with others, and letters of evaluation
- Evidence for the AAMC competencies that she has developed

The Experiences-Attributes-Metrics (EAM) model

Medical schools that are trained in the AAMC holistic review method will examine the applicant's experiences, attributes, and metrics to determine whether the applicant is a good fit for the school's class and mission.

Experiences include cultural, historical, world, and political events that have shaped the applicant's worldview, as well as life experiences, educational background, research experience, affiliations, community service, healthcare experience, leadership roles, and distance traveled.

Attributes include geography, ethnicity, gender identity, faith, family status, national origin, relationships, citizenships, sex, age, physical ability, race, sexual orientation, individual interests, fields of interest, intellectual curiosity, maturity, languages spoken, perspectives, leadership, values and beliefs.

Metrics include GPA, grade trends, and MCAT scores.

It's important for you and your premed to understand the holistic view of her life, personality, and path to medical school so she can write about it and talk about it clearly and with authenticity and passion with anyone and everyone she meets between now and matriculation to medical school. The personal statement and interview are opportunities for her to show what's important to her and how she interacts with the world around her. When she understands her narrative, she will be able to talk about herself in a mature and self-aware manner. The ability to convey her narrative will continue to serve her when she meets her classmates, connects with new mentors, and networks in the medical community.

Keeping a Notebook

From this point forward, it is critical that you and your premed both keep a dedicated notebook or document for writing down the inspiration, ideas, and stories developed in this section. I highly recommend the use of a cloud-based document from the beginning because your premed will be able to easily go back and add details, search for specific words, rearrange stories, or paste them into essays. Use headers for each section in your notebook and stay organized—it will be helpful to easily refer back to various sections when brainstorming for and writing the personal statement and secondary essays, and preparing for the interview.

When working through the brainstorming questions, both you and your premed should record your answers. You may remember events or stories in your premed's life that he has forgotten or passed by, or your unique perspective may shine light on qualities he doesn't recognize in himself. After your premed has built a collection of writings, he'll arrange it into a cohesive narrative and then revise it to bring out rich and interesting details. Sounds easy, yes? It is, if he keeps a notebook. And if he answers the questions you will guide him through with critically considered and thoroughly written responses.

When you are answering questions about your premed, consider the positive qualities other people have noticed in him. Look back at old narrative grade reports; think of comments made by teachers, coaches, and counselors that made you feel proud.

Daily Journaling Prompts for Your Applicant

Today as I worked in this lab and contemplated its relevance to my future in medicine….

- What surprised me? The answer shows us your mind and how it works.
- What touched me? The answer shows us your heart and how it responds to the human beings around you.
- What inspired me? The answer shows us your life purpose, the longing of your deepest inner soul, and how it is called to medicine

Conversing vs. Writing

Sometimes it's hard to get started writing. There are a few alternatives to sitting down at the computer to help get you and your premed started here. You can have a conversation about the following topics and questions, and answer them verbally. One of you should write or type the conversation, or you can have a third person be the transcriber. Or you can record the conversation digitally and listen to it later to transcribe it.

Mental and Emotional Preparation

There is a growing body of research and experience that confirms that meditation really does contribute to mental clarity, confidence, productivity, and a sense of wellbeing. So my recommendation is that you sit for 2 to 5 minutes before each counseling and writing session. Breathe deeply in and out, and concentrate on a positive affirmation such as, "I am writing about myself with curiosity and ease."

Building Evidence

What follows in this chapter is a long list of appreciative questions for you and your premed to answer about her unique qualities, ideas, and strengths. After developing a field of strengths, covering the areas that matter to medical schools (academics, service, understanding of clinical medicine, research and extracurricular initiatives, in that rank order) and that matter to your child, she will want to develop her evidence for those qualities. Evidence documents the strength. Medicine is evidence-based. Admissions committees speak the language of evidence.

For all answers, include a story about an event or experience that provides evidence for the specific answer. Get in the habit of writing three-sentence stories with a beginning, middle, and end sentence. Some stories will provide evidence for multiple questions. In that case, give the story a nickname so you can refer to it repeatedly. The stories that are referred to frequently may provide the foundation for your premed's personal statement. Here's an example:

My dad is a surgical oncologist, who had become progressively more bitter and disenchanted with medicine because "all his patients died anyway" and he wanted to quit. My mom went into labor in our apartment when I was 12 years old and I watched it progress so fast that my dad had to remember how to deliver a baby. When my newborn brother dropped into his arms and their eyes met for the first time, I saw my dad recover joy again in the skills he possessed.

Life Story

This is a fun and easy exercise that will build your premed's inventory of stories to choose from for the rest of the exercises in this section. Take as much time as you need to write down a list of notable and significant events and memories, starting at the beginning of your child's life. After the life story is complete, review the timeline to confirm that the following events are included, if they apply:

- Personal illness or injury
- Barriers in healthcare (socioeconomic or cultural)
- Foreign and domestic clinical experience
- Memorable interactions with doctors or patients
- Research and laboratory experience
- Teaching or mentoring experience
- Leadership experience
- Teamwork
- Public and community service
- Illness or death of a friend or family member
- Recovery of a friend or family member
- Challenges with the academic record
- Other academic pursuits
- Extracurricular activities
- Unique qualities

Background

Ask your premed to describe the following topics and then write one interesting three-sentence story related to each one.

- Cultural background
- Family structure

- Place you grew up
- Type of community you grew up in
- Occupations of your family income earners
- Siblings and their jobs
- Role models
- Hobbies or sports
- The world of medicine

World of Medicine

Ask your premed to reflect on his experience with the world of medicine by answering the following questions. Write a story that provides evidence for each answer.

- Why do you want to be a physician/dentist/health care professional?
- How are you making an informed choice about a life in medicine?
- What do you know about what it is like to be a patient, directly or indirectly?
- What appeals to you the most about being a doctor?
- What do you know about what it is like to be a physician?
- What current problems in the world of medicine do you think about?
- How do you want to make a difference in the world of medicine?
- What do you value in doctors?
- Have you combined your knowledge of medicine and another academic field to solve a problem?
- What do you want medical schools to know about you?
- Why do you belong in medicine?
- What experience made you feel really clearly that medicine was for you?
- What did you gain from research that will help you in medical school?
- Why is it important to integrate scientific understanding with a humanistic orientation to medicine?
- How do you envision using your own potential impact now and in the future, to learn more about this problem,

to address it, to raise awareness of it, and to ultimately contribute to the solution?

Personal Growth

With your premed, explore how they have grown from their experiences. Begin to articulate how they internalize experiences and move forward from them.

- How has your faith made you resilient and hopeful?
- What did you learn from adverse events? What were your coping skills and how did you bounce back? Explore family and friend dysfunction, illness, death, bad grades, depression, anxiety, distractions, diversions.
- When have you voluntarily interacted with others who were different from you?
- How did your inclusiveness affect you—and them?
- What life events or activities have changed you the most in the past 3-4 years? How have they changed you?
- If you could begin college again, what would you do differently? What would you do the same way again?
- When you have been faced with multiple demands, how have you managed priorities? How have you become better at this during your college years?
- How do you handle your mistakes or errors? How would you handle them in medical practice?
- How have you used lessons learned from your mentors?
- How have you grown and what have you learned about yourself and others through your relationships with your spouse and children, if you have your own family?

Contribution

Ask your applicant to examine what makes them unique and distinctive. They will eventually describe these qualities to the medical schools who ask them to express how they will contribute their diversity, experiences, and qualities to the medical school class and community.

- What do you value in yourself?

- What do you value in friends?
- What do you value in teachers?
- What do you value in a learning environment?
- How have you evolved?
- What is your purpose in life?
- What is your contribution to your world?
- How would your best friends describe you?
- What is your most important attribute?
- What can you say about yourself that your recommendation letters may not?
- What will you contribute to your medical school community?
- How have you impacted the lives of others?
- Are you community-oriented or globally-oriented?

Personal Strengths

You often feel tired, not because you've done too much, but because you've done too little of what sparks a light in you. ~Alexander Den Heijer

When I ask the applicant what they see as their strengths, I don't define a strength as something the person is good at. I define it rather as something that makes them feel strong when they do it. Helping others, fixing situations, doing "good" (benefit to others) and doing well (achievement: academic, research, job, for example) are all ways of exercising strengths. At this point, you want to name the strength. This is kind of like naming the baby.

- What personal qualities or skills make you feel strong, competent, and effective?
- What do you think you are best at of the activities you regularly do in your daily life?
- What are your strengths in academics, service, clinical medicine, and research?
- What drains you or do you have an aversion to, regardless of your skill at it?
- What do you think you are worst at of the activities you regularly do in your daily life?
- How do you try to overcome your weaknesses?

- What are your strengths of character?
- What are your strengths as a learner?
- How has your ability to learn grown and developed in and out of the classroom?
- What are your strengths as a leader?
- What are your strengths as a steward of the community?
- Are there strengths and talents that an admissions officer wouldn't realize from reading the rest of your application?

Questions to Ask Others

When your premed asks others about their views of them, they are seeking an outside perspective that can help them to be more self-aware when they write about themselves. Write down the exact words of the interview or record the conversation.

- What do others value about you?
- How do others rely on you?
- Have they seen you make a difference?
- What one thing would they change about you?
- Go over "36 Questions in Love," which you can find through an internet search. These questions were designed by a positive psychologist for people who are interested in finding companionate love in each other to pose and respond to. It's a great exercise for families who already love each other to do together at this critical phase in their premed's life.

Mapping Stories to Competencies

We discussed the professional competencies that medical school admissions officers use to assess applicants in an earlier chapter. A useful tool for translating the applicant's narrative stories into useful information for essays and interviews is a table that correlates each story to the competencies that were developed or strengthened from that experience. Here's an example:

Story/Experience	Competencies Developed
I helped bring my lab into compliance by researching compliance, developing protocols, training my colleagues, and submitting reports.	Teamwork, critical thinking, oral communication, reliability and dependability

Intentional Reflection

The narrative build process is the single most valuable part of my own system of advising. It reflects one of the greatest unanticipated long term benefits of applying to medical school: precious few young people ever find a period of time when they can deeply, honestly and positively reflect on who they really are, and how they got to the present moment in their lives. The narrative build grew out of nine years of composing committee letters for Cornell applicants. It grew out of me listening to admissions committee panels at conferences exhorting advisors to make sure that our students "understand their narrative!" I distinctly remember a highly accomplished premed who sat beside me at such a meeting, turning to me with a puzzled expression, and whispering: *What's a narrative?*

In preparing materials for hundreds of committee letters over a decade, I came to recognize that simple little acts have dropped out of modern life, such as writing weekly letters back home, one to your parents, one to a grandfather, one to your best friend from high school, acts that allowed us to process our life for a particular audience. Without these bygone rituals, our premeds and their friends sometimes do not know how to reflect, nor to articulate who they are with authenticity and conviction. The narrative build gives them a chance to do that, and it gives me a chance to get to know them and become deeply invested in serving their dreams. As they refer back to the narrative build during the application cycle and beyond, they are grateful for this "database of me." They continue to use it for interview preparation and even for residency applications. Parents love it as a snapshot of how their child has arrived in the adult world, ready to make an impact. I hope you enjoy doing this with your premed as much as I do with the ones who seek my guidance.

17 The Essays

Advice abounds on how to write great essays. We have our own tip sheet to guide your applicant through the process. Here, I focus on guiding you, the parent or counselor, through how to be the best support as your premed writes their personal statement, activities descriptions, most meaningful activities, and secondary application essays.

Think on this: What essential positive qualities have other people noticed in my kid? Look back at old narrative grade reports; think of comments made by teachers, coaches and counselors that made you feel proud. Write them all out. And while you are at it, think of what makes you proud. You may find it hard to distill these memories into words or themes that your premed will need to begin work. In this case, you can talk it over with someone who is intelligent about people, and develop your ideas.

With this superstructure in place, as you read or listen to your applicant's stories, think of how each one reveals her strengths. When she can relate the details of personal and professional growth and development that arose from her attributes and the experiences she chose, she will give meaning to her narrative and make it convincing.

Writing a Personal Statement

Timeframe of drafting: January through April

Timeframe of submitting: May, or with the primary application

Length: depends on specific primary application your applicant will be submitting

At the end of the primary application, there is an opportunity to make what is usually referred to in the application as "personal comments." This is the personal statement (PS), and your applicant will use it to give the application screener a few prime examples of stories that show who she really is; these give rich context and memorable details that do not fit into other parts of the application.

Because the personal statement is part of the most generic, centralized form of the application, and many different schools will evaluate it, it needs to fit the screening mindset of most, if not all the readers who will review it. Applicants often worry that this requirement will make it so their personal statement has to be rife with clichés, but avoiding that is a relatively easy fix.

Think of the personal statement as supporting the admissions selection process and establishing the applicant's narrative. While admissions committees place varying weight on this particular part of the application, they all want to learn more about who she really is and why she wants to study medicine. The personal statement is also evidence for the application process: it demonstrates her ability to reflect on her life with perspective and to communicate well in a written format.

This statement is actually a brief essay. It is neither the story of her life (autobiographical), the charmer's answer to "tell me about yourself," nor is it a narrative-form resumé of accomplishments. It's a place to share a story or two, and ideas about herself that highlight some of the competencies she has developed. Statements of this kind must be well-drafted and polished compositions that adhere to length and topical constraints. The goal is for the reader to develop an interest in the applicant, to take away a true sense of her authenticity and an impression that she is a worthy candidate who is ready for medical school.

How to Pick Stories for the Personal Statement

For the personal statement, usually two to three stories can fit in the 5300 characters (the AMCAS character limit) at most. Here is an example of a story that helped to reveal a lot about an applicant's strengths.

I volunteered as a Post-Anesthesia Care Unit waiting room liaison during the summer after my sophomore year. The families, furrowing their brows and wringing their hands, appeared as vulnerable as their loved ones undergoing surgery. After the operation, the surgeon would step into the waiting room, announce the family's name, and welcome them into the private conference room. The air was always thick with tension. But what could I do? A free cup of coffee, a banana nut muffin, and a pamphlet on "Family Visitation Rules & Guidelines" were the only things I could offer. In talking with several families, though, I discovered that their angst was directly attributed to the uncertainty of the clinical process: unexplained medical jargon, potential risks of surgery and medications, and concealed operating room activities. I shared these concerns with the PACU nurses and together we began providing expected timelines for visitation. By relaying this information to the families in the waiting room, I was moved by how the anxiety on their faces melted away.

Feeling more at ease, family members began sharing stories that evoked in me a profound respect for the strengths of humanity: the courage of a mother whose 3-year-old was undergoing a brain tumor resection, the faithfulness of four daughters coming from afar to care for their mother after spinal surgery, the selflessness of a nephew who donated his kidney to save his aunt's life. I originally volunteered as a waiting room liaison in order to gain experience interacting with patients and their families. By summer's end, I found myself inspired by these ordinary people who possessed an extraordinary devotion to their loved ones. My heart became set on a career in medicine to preserve the family ties they so cherished.
~Dr. David Ge

The personal statement is written from direct experience. Turning a richly felt inner experience into a polished outer form takes more time than you would ever want to plan for, and more humility regarding feedback than you thought you needed. It is worth every bit of that time. Most important, it helps your premed feel really good about herself during the often bruising application cycle. It's not uncommon during some of the tough, wait-it-out moments, months after the primary application has been submitted, for one of my applicants to say to me: *I love my personal statement. It's become a kind of security blanket for them.*

There are essentially two ways to develop the essential message that brings the personal statement alive: top down or bottom up. The bottom up method is typified by this actual conversation: *Honey, remember when you called me from the lab your freshman year? You were checking the electrode placements on mice one after another, when one stopped moving in your hand. You had just learned chest compression resuscitation in your EMT training and you did CPR on the mouse. It looked up at you, restored to life and you called us! Write about that, honey!* In other words, your applicant can start with your favorite story—or better, hers, and build the big message. That personal statement started with the sentence: "I will never forget the first life I saved."

The second way to develop the message is to spend time reflecting and conceptualizing, to articulate the themes and establish the structure of the statement before coming up with stories that provide evidence for those themes. Tools abound for wringing the true message out of the surrounding blah blah blah. You could have your premed go online to the website owned by Gallup, where it administers the CliftonStrengths assessment. I ask my applicants to take the Top 5 CliftonStrengths, and often, we find that the Top 5 strengths are recurring themes in their narrative. The score report of top strengths will prompt many thoughts about who they really are and the source of their interest in medicine. Another way is to write an elevator speech. Instructions for that also abound.

Rachel Naomi Remen (rachelremen.com) is a physician who works on issues of burnout and resilience. She has written two

NY Times bestsellers that relate stories she has gleaned from a life in medical environments. In these stories, one sees the inner qualities that physicians connect with to keep their spirits up about their work. You can read her work and see if you find your applicant in the stories. This will help you to point out their own life themes, how they might want to talk about them, and the life experiences that support them.

Reading the Personal Statement

Helping your premed choose from many stories is a great gift. You base the choice among anecdotes on a few criteria. Which ones are most compelling? Which ones really showcase the strengths? Do they give the sense of a drop in a stream of experience (plus) or do they stand as the only interesting thing that ever happened to your premed?

When you read stories, look for and ask for the details. Why did you do that? Who did you encounter/work with/or help? Why was it important to you? What did you learn? An important role of the advisor and editor is to help the applicant fill in the details of each story and articulate the observations, experiences, and actions that really inspired, touched, and motivated them.

Here is a list of questions you can ask your premed to help them move forward and through the personal statement, and include important details. Ask him to write the answer to questions you pose. His responses can result in a more natural feel to his language, as well as providing evidence for his assertions. Here are some good questions.

- What appeals to you the very most about being a doctor?
- What do you need the medical schools to know?
- Why do you belong in medicine?
- Would you tell me about a time when you felt really clearly that medicine was for you?
- What are your strengths as a learner? How has your ability to learn grown and developed in and out of the classroom?

- What are your strengths as a leader? What experiences have shown you that you have developed leadership skills?
- What are your strengths as a steward of the community? How did they develop?
- What did you gain from research that will help you in medical school?
- Tell me about someone else's work: a book, movie, quote, TV ad, show, anything you have read, listened to or watched in entirety, with all your attention, recently and how it has affected you?

What is the Theme?

There are many durable themes for personal statements: interdependence, integrity, compassion, problem solving, fear and courage, anger and joy, grief and passion, loss, faith, embracing otherness and common humanity, or cultural competence.

What is the one big picture question your applicant wants their statement to answer? Here are examples:

- How did I personally and intimately discover the power of becoming more culturally competent in my own life?
- What are my most formative and transformative moments as a person who promotes humanity in medicine?

If she comes up with several competing candidates for the big question, ask her to send them all to you after she has refined them a bit. Refining them means rewording them until she feels in her gut that, "YES! This is my question!" Not just that it sounds good. It has to feel that she owns this question in her body, heart, AND mind.

Writing the Activities Descriptions

Timeline: same as the personal statement, both will be submitted as part of the primary application

Length: depends on specific primary application your applicant will be submitting, but approximately 600-700 characters

In the primary application activity and experience section, your applicant will document all of the clinical, research, and community service engagements that have prepared him for medical school, but will have limited space to delve into them. This list of activities can be based on the applicant's resume, but it can also include activities of importance that would not necessarily be listed on a resume, such as playing Mahjong for ten years every Sunday with his grandmother and her friends. Research is the only academic-type experience that belongs in the list—not coursework. Do not cite high school activities, unless engagement continued after graduating from high school. The only departure from this would be if the applicant is lacking any service or clinical experiences in college or post-college, but they did something exceptionally noteworthy before college.

I suggest taking a journalistic approach to describe each activity: a narrative of the facts and why the applicant chose this activity. What exactly did he do, how was he involved, who else was involved, and what did he learn? The when and where details will be entered separately and don't necessarily need to be included in the description, since it can be a challenge to fit in all the details within the character limit anyway.

Information Needed for Each Experience

Experience Type:
Most Meaningful Experience: Yes or No (You can indicate yes to a max of 3/15)
Experience Name:
Dates:
Total Hours:

Contact Name & Title:
Contact Email:
Contact Phone:
Organization Name:
City / State / Country:
Experience Description:

- How much time did you spend and how often?
- What was your role and what were your responsibilities?
- Who else was involved?
- What did you accomplish?
- Did you make an impact?
- What qualities did you demonstrate or strengthen?
- How did you grow from this experience?

Most Meaningful Activity Essays

Only on the AMCAS application for allopathic medical schools, three of the activities will be designated by the applicant as "Most Meaningful." For these activities, an additional 1325-character essay will be required to discuss why it was important or meaningful (again, this is in addition to the shorter description mentioned above). AMCAS asks you to: "Consider the transformative nature of the experience, the impact you made while engaging in the activity, and the personal growth you experienced as a result of your participation." The applicant can answer questions like these as an approach to writing these shorter statements.

- How did I position myself or contribute?
- How did I learn from, blossom in, and make best use of my role in making the organization functional and good for everybody involved?
- How did I strengthen specific core competencies?
- What did I take away or how did I grow?
- How does this experience affect how I view medicine or plan to practice medicine?

- Do your three most meaningful essays, taken together, provide a holistic view of your core competencies, personal values, and motivations?

When reading through your applicant's most meaningful essays, think about these tones and descriptions: humility, mentorship, teamwork, mastery, authority, leadership, collaboration, scholarship.

For many applicants, one of their most meaningful experiences will be research. People often think about the internal workings of the lab as a kind of home base or family on a big campus. In the lab environment, they learn how productivity and scholarship are furthered by collaborative teamwork and mentorship. Sometimes, the hands-on and frontier or cutting edge aspects of research are meaningful. Sometimes, watching people attempt and fail and persist provides meaning. Often, just the culture of the lab and the interactions it evokes—real-time thinking out loud, watching your own ingenuity and others' in real time, knowing graduate students and postdocs and seeing their milieu and aspirations, as well as being a microcosm of diversity—are potentially meaningful things to mention.

Writing Secondary Application Essays

Timeframe of drafting: March through July

Timeframe of submitting: July through September

After the primary application is verified and accepted as complete by AMCAS or AACOMAS, the application will be forwarded to individual medical schools who will then either automatically send a secondary application to the applicant or screen the applicant before deciding to send the secondary application. Each school chooses which additional information they will ask for in their secondary application, and some schools don't require any additional information. The secondary applications may or may not change from year to year.

Since it is important to submit all applications as early as possible, we advise pre-writing the secondaries using last year's secondary prompts for that school. It should be easy to find this information online; the Savvy Premed and Prospective Doctor websites keep up-to-date lists of historical secondary prompts.

As you help your applicant develop their secondary essays, or review them, keep these important tips in mind: address the prompt and emphasize "fit." Read through the prompt completely and be sure that the response clearly answers all parts of the prompt.

The secondary essays should highlight your applicant's "fit" with each school. To make the case for fit, he needs to understand what he can contribute and what he wants in a medical school. The more specific he is, the better his chances. It's not random, it's strategic.

For each school, your applicant can complete this table to help him focus the content of his essays to emphasize fit and to help you review the essays with fit in mind. I recommend filling in the table below for each school and referring to this when writing essays for each school (it is also very helpful for anyone who is reviewing your applicant's essays), and throughout the entire application process (preparing for interviews and networking events, writing updates, etc.)

List three specific things you love about the school (e.g., programs, values, curriculum) and how you will contribute.

Essay editing is best done with an ear for the audience and a keen sense of the premed's themes. I have found it challenging to teach parents how to edit secondary essays with both these considerations in mind. The admissions offices want to hear certain ideas, values and outlooks expressed by the applicant through the lenses of their experience and character in order to decide to interview an applicant and over the years, I have learned these things, one at a time. However your premed decides to draft the essays, the best help you can be is to recall their stories, help them put those stories in the context of their themes, and sit with them as they get to the final draft, one person reading out loud, the other reading the text, to make sure there are no oversights or off-tone statements. This part of preparing applications is quite an endurance exam. Nurture patience, have chocolate close at hand, and pour on the love.

I can tell you from abundant personal experience, it can be agonizing, sometimes excruciating, to witness a premed struggle to express themselves over countless essays as the beautiful spring and summer pass them by. Keep in your mind, as I must, that your premed's sense of worth is enriched when they do the writing themselves. If they have to learn to write at this point, so be it. They must learn sometimes. Nurture your faith in your premed. Let them make their own mistakes and let their own voice shine through in their writing.

18 How Letters Support the Narrative

Think not just about how the world has happened to you, but how YOU have happened to the world.

~Mercedes Rivero, Assistant Dean of Admissions, Rutgers New Jersey Medical School

Medicine is evidence-based. Admissions committees pay attention to evidence more than promises. Letters of recommendation (LoR) are the evidence that documents your applicant's attributes and experiences. Premeds should not be passive about building relationships with potential letter writers, nor about the content of their letters, hoping that they will magically augment their narrative.

Letters are important to admissions committees because they are viewed as honest, accurate, revealing and significant. They provide authenticity to your applicant's own input and give the selection committee confidence in him. Letters corroborate his own statements about his interests and activities. Letters attest to his character. He cannot do that for himself.

An LoR writer will typically address these questions:

- How do I know this applicant? (Introduction)
- What is the nature of my observations of the applicant? (Body)
- How do I regard this applicant as a medical professional? (Conclusion)

When thinking about who to ask for a LoR, reflect on this list of questions. Professionals who taught, supervised, or collaborated with your premed are potential letter writers. Your premed can help their letter writer really get to know them by talking about things that surprise, touch, and inspire them. Earlier, we discussed how important it is for your applicant to pave the way for good letters through networking—and this is when those years of mindful networking really start to pay off. Your premed can reflect on their relationship with potential writers by considering:

- How does the writer view my degree of commitment to medicine?
- How does the writer view my potential to be an excellent doctor?
- How will I interact with the letter writer with authenticity and confidence?
- Does the letter writer know how and why the activity they are writing about connects to the rest of my narrative?

Your applicant is probably not the only person the letter-writer will be writing about. It is natural for writers to compare applicants to other students, past and present, when considering how to compose a letter. You can reflect together on the ways in which the letter writer will distinguish your applicant positively from other applicants.

Mechanics of Asking for a Letter

Timing of requesting LoRs depends on many individual factors. Your premed can ask before leaving a lab, or ending an activity or course, or wait to ask until important activities are near completion. They should not ask prematurely, just to suit checklist deadlines.

An applicant should ask the writer at least one month before the date that they have determined to be optimal for their application to be complete. The applicant should give the writer a specific deadline, usually a month from the date of the request, and ask permission to remind them about it.

Face-to-face asks are best. Second best is over a video conferencing application. Once the letter writer agrees, the applicant will need to ask if the writer can provide a strong LoR. The applicant can hand supplemental information to the writer when they ask, or follow up by email as soon as possible after the interaction to provide these materials. Occasionally, a letter-writer will even offer for the student to draft the LoR themselves!

Applicants should ensure that the writer knows that the letter must be on letterhead with the letter writer's signature. It can be signed manually, and scanned, or they can paste an electronic signature in the appropriate spot. If the letter writer does not understand this, your applicant's letter may be rejected by the school or its contents dismissed without the admissions office even notifying the applicant of this.

If an applicant must ask for a LoR by email, make sure that the last line contains a clear question that mandates a response. We all get a lot of email and it is easy to postpone reading it. By asking a question, you are more likely to get a response and to know that the potential writer understood the request. Applicants should not ask for an assurance of a strong letter by email–only in person. Applicants should follow up by phone meeting if the request was made by email. After the writer agrees, ask if they need more information and send an email with documents attached (discussed below).

Interfolio

I suggest that your premed register for an account at Interfolio, an online credentials storage service, and have their letter writers upload LoRs there. It's a great way to store letters and easily send them where they need to go. It gives you maximum control over letter distribution.

How to Support the Letter Writer

In order to get the best and most timely letters of recommendation, it's important to consider the writer's perspective. Letter writing takes time; the writer will face competing priorities, limited energy for writing, and competing motivations for how she wants to use her time. To assist the writer in expediting the letter request, applicants can support the composition process fully by providing information that will be needed for the letter, without giving the impression that their input might stain the integrity of the LoR.

Your applicant can create a stronger chance of selection when he makes his case clearly to the letter writer with evidence, so the letter will be grounded in the applicant's narrative and thus lend credibility to his application. Applicants should give the writer a well-written, clear and comprehensive supplemental information document to make their job faster and easier. The writer needs to address particular questions. Your applicant can help by answering these questions factually in a supportive document that they give the letter writer when they ask for the LoR.

Outline of a Letter of Recommendation

This is how a strong and comprehensive letter is typically formatted. In providing information for the writer, an applicant can write about the topics in paragraphs one, two, and three (the rest is up to the writer). IF the applicant is asked to draft the entire letter, touch on all of the topics below. Ask an advisor or editor to review the draft.

Paragraph 1: The relationship

How the letter writer knows the applicant, how long (in number of years, not "since 20xx"), nature of the relationship, and the generally favorable impression of the applicant.

Paragraph 2 and 3: Professional and personal qualities

The best or most significant skills, talents, behaviors, professional qualities, and competencies the applicant learned and demonstrated during their relationship with the letter writer.

The applicant can describe one or more anecdotes, projects, or initiatives they were involved with to illustrate their skills, talents, behaviors, professional qualities, and competencies. These descriptions should include:

- what their role was
- why it was an important and/or useful activity
- what their goals were and how they achieved them
- any challenges they met and/or overcame

The applicant should read the full AAMC Core Competencies and paste in the descriptions of the relevant competencies for each activity they describe so the letter writer can refer to the competencies for verbiage. Remember, competencies are the language of the admissions committee.

Paragraph 4: Potential as a doctor

How the applicant's skills, behaviors, and qualities relate to their potential to become what the writer considers a good doctor. (Evaluation of their cognitive, psychological (empathy, compassion) and communication skills.)

Paragraph 5: Summary

This paragraph can contain a final recommendation, comparative evaluation, or vote of confidence.

Research Letter from a Primary Investigator

Although your applicant can apply this information to any LoR, it is particularly important when they ask for a letter from someone they conducted research with, or a primary investigator (PI). When they discuss the letter with their PI, ask the PI to give a high assessment of them and to single them out: "This applicant stands out from others as a person who can make a contribution because (of the evidence they have provided to the PI)."

Applicants need to muster the confidence to ask for this. Again: the applicant needs to ask their PI to distinguish them positively from others, to rate them highly. The most comfortable and humble way to ask for this is to provide a concrete and well-documented (with detail) example of something that all colleagues agree the applicant did very well. The PI's words must show advocacy for the applicant's candidacy in the concluding paragraph of the letter. This letter must make the applicant stand out as a person who can make a contribution.

Great letters make successful applicants to medical school. It is easy to be passive and to trust the letter writer to compose the letter, but I urge you to encourage your premed to prepare the ground for the letter writer. This is work and can feel, like other aspects of the application process, unpleasantly self-serving. Nevertheless, there is no time like this one to break through resistance and reframe the whole task. Writing letters takes a lot of time and making them sound good takes more time. If the premed prepares thoughtful, brief, usable material that jogs the memory of the letter writer and makes the content expression easy, the letter writer will be grateful that your premed saved them time. The time they saved will be used in writing glowing adjectives to describe your premed, which will help to further their application at the medical schools. As a parent, busy yourself, you can encourage this and proofread the materials. This will be a great gift to your premed and the person who is professionally supporting their progress toward their dream.

19 Making A School List

Before submitting any application, your premed needs to think about whether they are applying to osteopathic and/or allopathic medical schools, and whether they want a combined degree (MD+ MPH, MBA, or JD), because the application may be different for these programs. Beyond that, your premed must choose the schools where they can see themselves thriving for the next four years.

Osteopathic vs. Allopathic

When you talk with your premed, recognize that osteopathic schools exist under a completely false stigma–completely. It's a stigma that was created by politics and lobbying to spread the idea that osteopathic schools were not high quality, but it's false. Essentially the stigma is now based on entrance requirements and it kind of goes along with the old adage, "I would never join a club that would lower itself to accept me." Osteopathic schools have a much greater range of MCAT scores than allopathic schools, which results in lower average MCAT metrics for accepted students. Their average GPAs are often just as high as allopathic medical schools. They don't go into the stratosphere of 3.9, but they definitely go into the 3.7 category.

Admissions offices at osteopathic schools take a pass-fail approach to MCAT scores. They don't necessarily think that a higher MCAT score means an applicant is more able or suitable for medicine. They don't want someone coming to osteopathic school who doesn't understand and fully appreciate the osteopathic health and healing philosophy, which includes a lot more about preventative medicine, the interconnectedness of body systems, as well as Osteopathic Manipulative Treatment (OMT), a hands-on practice of moving a patient's muscles and joints by stretching or applying gentle pressure.

Osteopathic medical training is based on a musculoskeletal understanding that is likely to be greater than allopathic students gain because osteopathic physicians must recognize and feel the muscles, nerves and bones from outside of the body. Your student should apply to osteopathic medical school to receive a DO degree if they want to do a more holistic form of doctoring or really learn how to do primary care, or conduct research that is more directed at understanding the interconnected nature of the body. Osteopathic schools often have lower tuition, smaller class sizes, and consider themselves every bit equal to any allopathic school.

It used to be harder for osteopathic physicians to get residency matches than it was for allopathic physicians, because there was a higher bar for them compared to allopathic medical graduates. They had to prepare for and pass two different licensing exams. Since the most common residency match is now combined for osteopathic and allopathic medical graduates, osteopathic physicians face fewer barriers and any one person can overcome all of it to land the residency match they desire.

As a very general rule, if a student has below a 3.6 GPA and 510 on the MCAT, they should apply to both osteopathic and allopathic schools, to increase their chance of acceptance by the end of the cycle. One important thing to note about osteopathic schools is that their admissions cycle is not as time-sensitive as the AMCAS application cycle. Your applicant can apply a little later and should if they are applying to MD and to DO schools. When an applicant is accepted at an osteopathic school, they are asked to pay a deposit ranging from $500 to $2,500. Often this is non-refundable, unfortunately. As a practice, this can become costly if your applicant is on a waitlist and the school is not their top choice, but it's currently their only choice. Do you put down the money and possibly forfeit it if they choose to go to a different school later in the cycle? It can be an expensive decision.

School Research and Comparison

Applicants should research and consider multiple factors when deciding where to apply. While you or your premed can start compiling this research into a spreadsheet in the spring, a good time to settle the school list is after submitting the primary application and before receiving secondary applications. Applicants only need to list one school to submit the AMCAS primary application to begin transcript verification, and they can add more before verified applications are sent to medical schools at the end of June. The osteopathic application service is AACOMAS and the allopathic is AMCAS. There is a different service for Texas medical schools: TMDSAS, which includes the DO, MD and DDS (dental schools) in that state.

Applicants can set up a Google Drive-based spreadsheet to note their research. This is a valuable tool for school choice. It is useful throughout the cycle, writing secondaries, preparing for interviews and updating schools when they make the case for their fit for the school.

Here are the most commonly used criteria. When you set up the spreadsheet, rank order them from most to least important, placing the most important farthest to the left of the columns.

Rural/Urban

Proximity to home

Tuition and Financial Aid

Curriculum

MCAT/GPA targets

Mentoring and support programs

Class size

Residency outlook

Distinctive school features

Early or innovative clinical/patient exposure

Faculty commitment to individuals

Well-structured student support system with ample communication on ongoing student opportunities / initiatives

Careers in medicine programming

Is the administration receptive to student feedback?

Does the school have rich resources to prepare you for the future healthcare environment?

Location – Is it rural or urban? Is it close to family or friends? Is it near a patient population of interest? Are there any other important factors related to location?

Tuition and Financial Aid – What are the costs and what is the potential for financial aid?

Financial aid varies incredibly – some medical schools give 100% of students free tuition and load on hidden fees that can amount to 20k a year, others may cover a standard tuition discount for their students. Some schools are committed to need-based aid only. Unfortunately, even if your premed is now approaching 30 and they have been financially independent for several years, the medical schools still base the provision of financial aid partly on parental assets and income. And then there is the Uniformed Services University of the Health Sciences, which is run by the United States. For students accepted at that medical school, the first year there's no tuition, they get paid to be an officer and their salary increases each year.

Curriculum – Is it lecture, problem-based learning, flipped classroom, body system-based, block scheduling, or something else? What is the grading system? Is the curriculum flexible? What electives, research, and other learning opportunities are there?

Metrics – What is the school ranking? What are its median MCAT and GPA for accepted students? What is the acceptance rate for In-State vs Out-of-State applicants?

Mentoring and support programs – Is the class size conducive to close relationships with mentors? Are academic and career advising structured or unstructured? Does the school foster a collaborative culture?

The mentoring culture is very important. Mentoring culture in a school really depends on how faculty are treated and how seriously the school treats the goal of recruiting a diverse faculty. The more diverse the faculty, the more different kinds of people your medical student can go to for guidance. It's really hard being a woman in medical school when all faculty members are men. Very few women and minorities find mentoring without searching for it. Encourage your student to find out what the identity makeup of faculty is and if mentorship is structured and flexible. A structured mentorship culture that is flexible allows a student to choose the right mentors. Mentorship culture also includes high quality, individualized and accessible academic and career advising.

Residency outlook – Before choosing a medical school, it is a good idea for your applicant to feel confident in their chances to match into a residency they want. Look at the residency match list of the school on their website. If a school doesn't have the list on their website, it's a strong sign that they may not want to promote it. However, there are certainly exceptions. Some really great schools have surprisingly outmoded, outdated and incomplete websites.

Distinctive school features – Is the administration receptive to student feedback? Are students prepared for the future healthcare environment? Are there research or travel opportunities? What are the opportunities for early clinical/patient exposure, or to engage with the community? What options exist for interdisciplinary research or interprofessional learning? How is the work/life balance of students relative to other schools?

Stay Organized

Your premed should keep a well-organized spreadsheet with all of this information for each school. If it is hard to find this information online, call the admissions office. They exist to inform and recruit prospective students, as well as admit them!

Finally, consider and enter into the spreadsheet the following information, because it will provide content for secondary applications and interviews.

- What is the school's mission, vision, and diversity statement?
- What qualities does the premed have that align with the school's mission statement?
- What aspects of the school excite the premed the most?
- How will the premed use the opportunities offered by the school?

Realistic School Choice Lists

After consideration of all the factors that go into being happy and flourishing academically in medical school, consider some simple facts. It is easier to get into the premed's home state school than a state school in another state. It is easier to get into a school in the same state as the one where the premed went to college. Pick schools that have a higher probability of admitting your premed strictly for those reasons and keep them on the list. If your premed works for a medical school, put that one on the list. Finally, the premed should draw up a list of ten dream schools. Then they should justify why, besides an illustrious name, those are their dream schools, because they will need to make the case. Just because we have heard of a school and know it is prestigious does not mean it is the best school for our premed, for all the reasons in this chapter and many more. Once they have a good reason why, or even if they don't and they just want to try, then they should apply to those schools. I think most advisors recommend applying to 15-20 schools, but that varies dramatically. In general, if your home state is California or in the Northeast, I would apply to more, because the competition is exceptionally stiff for those premed applicants.

I will close with a fond memory of an applicant with whom I stay close. He was an international student from a Baltic country who had earned everything he ever received. His dad was a florist and his mom a nurse. He had an identical twin. After the two boys spent a year at a home stay in the US, they decided they wanted to go to US schools for college and medical school. Their parents told them that they could only afford to lose one of their sons and support only one leaving the country, and they would have to choose who would go. My applicant was obviously the one the twins chose.

He was accepted at many medical schools, including Columbia and Yale. He had trouble deciding because he and I thought Yale was a better choice, but his dad, who had sacrificed so much, wanted him to attend Columbia. He wanted to honor his dad. I found the dad's position curious. In the end, my applicant chose Yale, and at his college graduation, I had the pleasure to meet his parents, who spoke no English, for coffee. I asked my applicant to ask his father to explain to me why he had been so set on Columbia. The translated answer came back.

His dad replied, memorably: *Who ever heard of Yale University?*

20 Interviewing

How do I love thee? Let me count the ways...

~Elizabeth Barrett Browning (Sonnet 43)

Medical schools conduct interviews because they need to differentiate candidates who look equally strong on the application AND they want to recruit applicants who will have to choose between schools, to choose them. A study of admissions officers reported four purposes: verify information in the written application, gather additional information, make judgments and decisions, and recruit applicants. Every school has a fit agenda, which they use to decide how to fill their class. They consider:

- state residency
- MCAT quotas
- relationships with the school
- primary care vs academic medicine orientation
- idiosyncratic diversity goals
- particular personality types
- family connections to the area (not favoritism-based)
- school articulation agreements
- and more recently, commitment to social justice

Going into the medical school interview, there are three topics that your premed will need to be very familiar with and comfortable talking about—himself, the medical school, and health care. One of the goals of the interview is to show that he can build a warm connection with his interviewer. During his interview, your premed should definitely be himself, highlight his beautiful personality and sharp skills, and share his dreams. After your premed receives an interview invitation, the medical school will send information about the format of interview day and potentially even who will be conducting the interviews.

Different Types of Interviews

- Unstructured – Unstructured interviews are more personal to the interviewer and tend to be more unpredictable or unexpected in content. Unstructured interviews rely on the applicant to establish rapport over 30 minutes to an hour of conversation. The point is to emerge with an admissions committee member who is motivated to advocate for you.
- Structured – Structured interviews fall on a continuum from providing a set of questions interviewers are mandated to ask, to using the AAMC personal competencies to set up questions. Structured interviews allow the school to rationally and directly connect its mission and vision statement to the applicant, looking for a fit. Structured interviews are an attempt to eliminate subjectivity, unfairness, and elitism in the medical student selection process.
- Multiple mini interview (MMI) – A type of structured interview that consists of a series of situational judgement, scenario, and personal questions that the applicant has a few minutes to contemplate and a few minutes to answer, each in front of a different interviewer. All applicants are evaluated based on their answers to the same questions. Interviewers and candidates experience it as fairer than other interview models and it has proven to be a reliable predictor of clinical exam results in the third and fourth year of medical school.

- Extended interview with standard questions – This is designed to make the interview more objective, as all applicants give responses to the same questions and their responses can be compared to one another.
- Hybrids of the above

Interviewer bias has been shown to inflate the significance of non-academic experiences of high MCAT/GPA candidates. Medical schools address this by conducting "blind interviews" where the interviewer has not seen any of the application materials submitted by the applicant. Other times, the interviewer has some parts of the application, and some sections are held back to reduce interviewer bias. Applicants can ask at the admissions Q&A, or ask interviewers what they have reviewed of the application materials to strategize how to highlight their strengths and the evidence for them.

As interviews tend to be virtual since the pandemic, interview day might also include webinars on financial aid and special programs, panels, group discussions, additional writing or team activities, and conversations with current students.

Family Support with Interviews

A common mindset toward the interviewer is: *I want you to like me. How can I please you? How can I win you over?* All this self-revolving brain noise obscures the possibility that all the interviewer actually needs and wants, on the most essential human-to-human level, is to feel accepted by the person they are talking with. We are conditioned to hold back our own acceptance until we feel accepted by others. To overcome this conditioning, which is often unconscious, ask your applicant to think about how they would walk into the room of one of their sick patients to administer treatment. They would walk in with this mindset: *You are in good hands. My training allows me to be a good doctor for you. I really care about you and the outcome of this treatment.* This is how your applicant should walk into the interview room. They must show that they have faith in themself in a way that will encourage the patient or interviewer to have faith in them.

Review the school's mission statement and talk with your premed about why they are a good fit with the school—do this often! Start having practice interview conversations well in advance of the interview. Review their personal statement and secondary essays and generate questions that the interviewer may ask, such as, "Why did you do X activity? What did you learn from it? Tell me about Y." It can also be helpful for premeds to practice interviewing together—we encourage this a lot at The Mentoring Alliance and playing both roles, as interviewer and interviewee, provides insight for premeds preparing for their interviews.

Have your applicant write down ten reasons why they were invited to interview, from the most obvious to the least, from what the school already knows about them to what they need to know.

Use this list of the top 10 questions to prepare for. Your premed should write down the points they want to make for these questions and assign each to a finger on their hands to help them remember to hit on all the points during the interview. They should not memorize their responses word-for-word.

- Tell me about yourself. TIPS: The response can be either chronological, with high points, OR cite three strengths, with examples from the applicant's life history, OR describe what role the applicant appreciates playing most in another person's life and what role other people play in their life, with evidence.
- Why do you want to be a doctor and practice medicine? What is your understanding of the patient population and patient needs served by the medical school where you are interviewing?
- What programs and research at this school interest you?
- What are three or more ways that you fit/resonate/or uphold the school's mission statement?
- How will you add diversity to your class?
- What recent accolades have the school and its faculty or students received?

- What questions do you have for your interviewer about the school? Applicants should be prepared with questions for the interviewer. This is a must to further emphasize their interest in the school and to keep the conversation going.

Your role, as you listen to your applicant's responses is to give them gentle, but honest feedback. Consider the following:

- Do they respond in an informed, authentic manner—about themself, the school, and the field of medicine—that inspires your confidence in them?
- Is their response succinct but thorough, and not too long that it gets boring or hard to follow?
- Do they use interesting anecdotes from their life experience to illustrate their point?
- Do their responses align with or provide evidence for their themes and narrative?

Finally, for a virtual interview, ensure that your applicant has a good video camera, good lighting, and a neat background. There are many videos and articles about how to look good on a virtual conference call or interview. For an in-person interview, I recommend business attire with a distinctive and colorful scarf, earrings, tie, or bow tie.

Reading List for Your Applicant

Read articles and listen to podcasts by doctors about how healthcare issues and patient situations affect their daily practice. This content will help them bring up topics that an interviewer may relate to instantly.

Read books and articles by physician-authors such as Atul Gawande, Jerome Groopman, Abraham Verghese, Danielle Ofri, Rachel Naomi Remen, Paul Kalanithi, Perri Klass, Rachel Pearson and Paul Farmer.

Problems to Watch For and Work On

During interview practice, your applicant needs to be conscious of how they are presenting—you can help them by being an impartial observer and reflecting back to them what you observe. Your applicant can consider tweaking a few involuntary personality traits if they might end up rubbing the interviewer the wrong way. There are a variety of ways that the interviewer may perceive your applicant that will sabotage the interview:

- The interviewer didn't feel liked or respected.
- The applicant seemed overly rehearsed or scripted, with canned, prepared answers.
- The applicant could not produce substantive examples or evidence of skills or attributes she claimed to have gained or developed.
- The applicant seemed uninterested in questions if they weren't about their experiences or fit for medical school, such as hypothetical clinical scenarios or questions about problems in the healthcare system.
- The applicant seemed immature: giggling, not being able to think out loud about issues, playing with hair or other objects with their hands, inappropriate clothing, makeup, grooming, using typical adolescent vocal expressions (uptalk, vocal gravel, like-like-like), answering questions using personal or interpersonal situations with friends instead of professional roles and situations.
- The applicant was defensive.
- The applicant seemed self-centered: focused on their achievements instead of helping others and finding solutions.

Read up or watch TED talks about interviewing, body language, and connecting with other people. Notice your applicant's mannerisms and body language—preferably months in advance of the interview. Ask them if you can talk about any mannerisms that should be worked on. How do they want to show up on interview day? Come up with a plan to work through these issues.

The Ideal Interview

Whether the interviewer is blind to the application, partially blind or has reviewed it all, the interviewer asks thoughtful questions and gives the applicant a chance to autonomously build on her responses and fully address the prompt, question, situation or idea. When asked challenging questions—or questions about challenges and weaknesses—the applicant is given a chance to provide a complete answer and receive validation from the interviewer that he is satisfied with their response. The applicant can expect to feel that she got a fair chance to present her candidacy in person. If she is as good a fit for the school as the admissions committee thought she was when they extended the interview, she can expect to be given the chance to confirm their initial confidence with her. When your applicant exits the interview, she should feel better than when she walked in.

Take Notes After the Interview

After the interview, the premed needs to debrief by just writing everything that happened, everything they thought and felt, ways they did not feel good and what prompted that, and every other thought they have about how to improve next time. It is good for them to go over these notes with you. It is good for you just to listen with openness and curiosity as they sort things out.

Send Thank You Notes

It is polite to send a note to the admissions office at the school thanking them for the opportunity to interview, as well as to individual interviewers to reinforce the connection your applicant began to build on interview day. Some admissions officers may gently discourage thank you notes at the end of interview day, which is their way of subtly signaling to applicants that they won't make any difference to their candidacy. I advise sending thank you notes to interviewers anyway. Advise your applicant not to send the **same** thank you letter to the committee and the interviewer, as they are likely to both show up in the applicant file. They should send individualized letters to each person, commenting on a shared connection point during the interview. If your interview day was all MMIs, no thank you note is appropriate, as you have only brief interactions with them, but it is welcome to send a message to the people at the admissions office and let them know you felt welcomed and that you appreciated their organizational skill in making the day easy to navigate as an applicant.

Adverse Interviews

Usually, applicants feel relief after an interview, like they accomplished the next feat in their journey to medical school. But sometimes an interview will feel like it went wrong, or something just didn't feel okay or normal about it—it could be an adverse interview. Your applicant may exit thinking and feeling that their expectations for a complete, fair or impartial review were not met. They may doubt that the interviewer supports their candidacy. When your applicant experiences this, it's best to discuss with an advisor as soon as possible.

More often than I would like to remember, I have received an urgent text message from a restroom stall right after an adverse interview. Sometimes an applicant gets rhetorically cornered into making a naïve stand that the interviewer considers a red flag. There can be misunderstandings. Sometimes interviewers are known cannons (unintentional bullies or unconscious perpetrators of implicit bias) and the only recourse to be fair to the applicant is for the admissions committee to add more information to the file to make a better decision.

Reasons to Report the Adverse Interview

Be open to the possibility that the interview was just tough and the interviewer wanted to challenge the applicant. They could have written a glowing review afterward. After considering this possibility, and in consultation with an advisor, here are some reasons that your applicant may want to report the interview as adverse to the admissions office.

- She sensed implicit or explicit bias. Examples of this include questions that touch on stereotypes about ethnicity, gender or another essential attribute. For example, two Asian American women at one school were asked what they thought of the tendency for undergraduate Asian Americans to "self-segregate."

- The interviewer praised her, even effusively, but wanted to talk about something other than her candidacy. For example, an interviewer asked an applicant to explain his entrepreneurial family's successful business model. Another told an applicant at the outset that she would receive his highest marks for the interview and wanted to spend their time together talking over how he might help his daughter get into the applicant's prestigious undergraduate school.
- The interviewer was late, distracted, disorganized, apologized for not reading the file when he was expected to, or seemed to think the applicant was someone else entirely.
- She just felt weird after the interview and was unable to strike up anything resembling a natural conversation. Think about why that was, and if it was partly her responsibility, make sure to include that in any request for another interview.

How to Report an Adverse Interview

The first thing to address is: What happened? When your applicant tells you what happened, write it all down, or voice record it, or ask them to sit down immediately and write out everything. Review it all: the good stuff as well as the discomfiting moments. Balanced reporting gives whoever guides you through the aftermath a chance to sift through the experience and detect the elements that may make it worth reporting to the admissions office in the hope of giving the applicant a second chance. In other words, start with the subjective experience and work toward an objective focus.

Your applicant will need to make a swift decision to report the adverse interview to the Director of Admissions or the Chair of the Admissions Committee—usually the Associate Dean for Admissions—within two business days of the interview.

Consider it an incident report, not a complaint, and ask for a telephone call. Don't put everything in an email; the applicant needs to show that she can conduct a serious conversation in real time, and because the admissions official may have some input that will change the context of the situation. Your applicant should then try to depict the interview as it transpired, indicating where it became adverse and sharing candidly how she felt at various points, and how her feelings changed.

Requesting Another Interview

Remember that when you report a problem, you need to be prepared **to request a solution**. The only solution that can really change what happened is for your applicant to be offered a new interview. If she is not offered a new interview, it is likely that the admissions office has determined that the interviewer's rating did not adversely affect her candidacy. Trust them on that.

In the rare case that the person to whom your applicant reports the incident leaves her feeling that they treated her or her concerns in a demeaning or condescending manner, she may need to appeal to another person who has greater decision-making power. This is rare. The only reason I mention it is so you know that you can appeal.

If the interview was truly unfair or biased, in nearly all cases the admissions office will want to give the applicant another chance without any negative repercussions.

Recipe for a Great Interview

There are three states of being you can practice with your premed to prepare them for their interviews:

- Presence: Reside in the moment. When you find your attention slipping while speaking to someone, refocus by centering yourself.
- Power: Break down self-doubt. Tell yourself you are a doctor. You belong. Lift the self-stigmatizing thought that you are not enough. Impostor syndrome is the fear

that you're not worthy of the position you want. It only gets stronger as you go higher, so learn to deal with it now.

- Warmth: Radiate kindness and acceptance to everyone. It's the feeling you get from a close relative or a dear friend. During a virtual interview, I recommend that applicants tape the picture of someone who raises their endorphins next to the camera. Think: Why do I love you so much?

21 Updating Schools

The admissions cycle proceeds in fits and starts. You don't hear anything in June, not much in July. Action picks up for some in August, but mostly invitations are sent in September, October and November. In December, things quiet down. Invitations will pick up in January, but after that, in February and March, interview invitations are few and far between.

Waiting is hard. Encourage your applicant to spend the wait time connecting with their growing network—and preparing update letters. Concerted, well-organized follow up action is part of the admissions process. When an applicant continues to connect with medical schools in meaningful ways on a regular basis, they help the admissions staff to form a holistic view of them as a candidate. Showing schools that they are enthusiastic about becoming a student there AND a good fit can help them get interviews. Updates are recommended for any applicant who has not yet received an acceptance.

Updates consist of contact with people at the school, in the form of phone calls and/or letters from the applicant, or by others regarding the applicant, as permitted by the school. Applicants send them to maintain relationships with medical schools. It's best when the topics the applicant writes about are actually updates—new developments in their candidacy. They can also send things that reflect common interests they hold with the school. Whatever the content of the letter is, they must stay in touch to the degree that each school affords or welcomes. If schools prohibit updates, it's good to know that at the outset so the applicant can pack more information into the secondary application, if possible.

Types of Update Letters

Updates consist of directly informing schools of new information about the applicant or securing supplemental recommendation letters. A good update letter has substance and brevity. The content has to be about the applicant and their fit with the medical school. The point of the update letter is that the people who read it will remember the applicant, in a good way. Sometimes applicants feel that they have nothing new to offer. This is usually not true. There are subtle changes and growth going on in us all the time. If we pay attention, we will see them.

If they have had an interview, applicants can maintain their relationship with their interviewer—the person who will advocate for them in front of the committee—by sending letters about specific topics discussed during the interview, things the applicant learned about them, the applicant's fit with the school and new activities, experiences and interactions that have happened since the interview.

Your applicant can send letters to the committee to clarify old matters and introduce new things. The letter can reiterate commitment to the school, interest in certain programs, and the applicant's status if they have not received any interviews or acceptances.

Your applicant can request a new letter of recommendation that adds to what the committee already knows. A PI or supervisor can write a new letter noting accomplishments since their first letter. These letters often cover a specific time span after your applicant applied or interviewed. Additional letters of recommendation can really help your applicant's candidacy.

The applicant can drop short messages to the admissions office stating that they are still looking forward to hearing the admissions decision and they have not decided where they will go to medical school. One way to freshen up correspondence is to alternate messages—with one explaining personal reasons for wanting to attend (geographic proximity, for example) and the next explaining more professional reasons (curriculum, for example). Letters and phone calls from supporters are also perfectly reasonable methods to entertain in developing an update strategy.

Make A Plan

Help your applicant take stock of what has changed since they submitted applications and then figure out how to articulate what is new and substantive in their candidacy. As I discussed at length in another chapter, it is important to start planning continued professional development at least in the spring before the application is submitted, so that the applicant will have compelling information with which to update. Your applicant can pursue a new service or extracurricular activity to show how they are developing as a candidate. They can become involved with a project that shows how they can see a problem, mobilize their strengths and resources to solve the problem, and institute an innovative solution.

In updates, they can note accomplishments that show productivity and collaboration. Identify activities where your applicant has expanded their leadership skills. How else have they personally or professionally developed?

Remember to keep a tracking sheet of communications, with detailed notes on every action and interaction. Decide what the next follow-up is as soon as an action is completed. Pick a deadline for the next update. After three follow-ups, decide what is next in the strategy to get interviews—do they need a new letter? A change of strategy? To change the mode of communication?

Refer to the blog at premedadvisor.com for more advice about the best times to send updates to schools.

Continue Networking

Seeking and establishing connections is at the heart of how to improve the chances to get into medical school. Think of any contact you have who may have a connection with any of the schools where your applicant applied. Ask your friends, family, and colleagues if they know anyone with a connection. Your applicant can call or meet with the contact to speak with them about their career, their advice, and their candidacy and interests. The contact may be able to call the school of interest or send a letter to the admissions office.

Keep Up Morale

Refer to our earlier chapter again for advice on how to communicate with your applicant during these tough and trying times. For applicants, it can feel exhausting, stressful, or downright unnatural to compose and send these updates. Psychologically, it's reasonable that they would feel some things about the medical school admissions process that they don't want to share, like anger or resentment, or even a loss of self-worth. They might feel like they are losing all dignity and are begging. If they are offered or seek the assistance of any influential people, that might even accentuate their sense of not being good enough just on their own merits.

As the parent, you can listen when these feelings arise. Eventually, you and your applicant can confirm that they are not true. Your future doctor will contribute greatly to the health of countless people throughout their lifetime. Medicine needs them.

22 Accepted! Choosing The School

On the great day when your premed is accepted to medical school, it is indeed time for a celebration. Nothing makes my day shine like the text message: *I got into medical school! I am going to be a doctor!* While you are so happy for them, take a few minutes to feel really proud of yourself. You were along for the ride, but you made it so much smoother. Congratulations, from one proud advisor to one proud family.

Making Choices

When an applicant is accepted to medical school, they are asked to pay a deposit, which is almost always refundable when it is for allopathic medical schools and usually non-refundable and more expensive for osteopathic schools. I am invariably asked: *Does this mean I'm committing to the school?* The answer is no: it doesn't mean that. It just means that you're putting down a deposit and showing that you're interested. It is just a formality. However, a large deposit at an osteopathic school can force you to make an adverse decision from an economic standpoint, because the applicant may want to wait for schools that have placed them on alternate lists. Do you make the deposit and risk losing money if your applicant decides to go somewhere else, or do you pass up the acceptance?

As your applicant is accepted to medical schools, they will need to pay close attention to the deadlines and requirements of each school. For allopathic schools, there's the Choose Your Medical School tool on the AAMC website, that AAMC has devised to make sure every medical school has ample opportunity to precisely fill its class each year. The tool ushers applicants through a progressive tightening of their school choices. It begins with allowing the applicant to hold only three acceptances and giving up the rest. Since fewer than 5% of all applicants get into more than 3 schools, you are in good company if this doesn't affect you. The next step, later still, urges applicants to hold only one acceptance where they "plan to apply," but allows them to stay on waitlists. Finally, students are strongly urged to commit to one school by certain dates that each school specifies. This feels binding because you are asked to give up all your alternate lists.

The truth is that the schools want you and urge you to follow these guidelines, but unless the individual school specifically states that you will lose your acceptance if you do not abide by the protocols, these really are guidelines, not ultimatums. You can call and ask for wiggle room and they can agree or not, depending on your reason. Dates for each step of the Choose Your Medical School tool change on an annual basis. In the beginning of this process, all dates for decisions are the same for each school, but as we get closer to the end of the application cycle, each school has different dates of which potential matriculants are informed. Schools need applicants to adhere to the guidelines dictated by the Choose Your Medical School tool, but I think it's important to note that they are not legal mandates.

Nevertheless, at the end of the cycle, your applicant may need to decide if they are going to wait for an acceptance off a waitlist or go where they are accepted. They will need to find housing, which will get harder to find closer to the beginning of the school year. If they are accepted at a school where housing is scarce or expensive, or student housing is limited, that is a reason to just go with that school instead of waiting.

Additionally, if your premed is on a waitlist, it feels very precarious to look for apartments they may not need. The premed needs to have really good reasons for deciding to wait for a spot off that waitlist as the first day of orientation approaches.

If your applicant gets into multiple schools, they need to ask a couple of critical questions:

1. How important is it for them to be physically proximate to someone else? It could be you, it could be their significant other, it could be a friend or family member.
2. What's the difference in cost? If they want to go to a more expensive school, is it worth it?
3. What is the mentorship culture?
4. How does the school support student wellness?

Don't forget that the cost of living around the school is a major factor to consider. For example, it is cheaper to live in Worcester, MA than in central Boston, one hour away. Many schools that are in expensive urban areas have housing for their students, like Icahn School of Medicine at Mount Sinai in New York City and University of California San Francisco (UCSF) School of Medicine. One problem with living in student housing, as opposed to renting an apartment off campus, is that if your medical student needs to take a leave of absence from the school, they won't be allowed to remain in student housing. When students have mental problems and are counseled to take a break, this means that they become homeless at an already vulnerable time.

Naturally, financial aid is a factor in something as pricey as medical school. Schools that accept an applicant outright are more likely to give financial aid, while schools that accept an applicant off of waitlists have often used up their financial aid by the time they do. It's important to take into consideration the cost of tuition and any other fees, which can come as a surprise and add up. Almost everyone who goes to medical school takes out loans. If a parent can afford to subsidize their premed's medical education in any way, the number one way to do so is to pay interest on their student loans. Your payment of the annual interest of 6% now will eliminate the compound interest accumulating every year of medical school. For them to pay compound interest every year becomes a much bigger debt.

In Case of Disagreement

Parents need to know that even if they are familiar with the name of a school, it doesn't mean it's a good school for their student. If you and your premed disagree about where they should go to medical school, each of you should draw up a list of criteria you are using to make that decision. And then you should each rank both lists of criteria from most important to least important and have a discussion. Then you'll see where the disagreement is.

Let's say you are from Texas and your premed gets into a University of Texas medical school, which means a considerably subsidized tuition, and they also get into the University of Illinois Chicago School of Medicine and they want to go there because they don't want to be far from their fiancé. But UIC tuition may be three, even four times the price of the UT school and they may not be able to become an in-state student there to reduce the costs. You, the parent, want to be close to them to support them. They want to go to school near their partner. Let them go. If you have the means and the motivation to contribute to their medical education, you could offer to pay the same amount as the Texas tuition, and leave it to them to do the math.

After Committing to Enroll

When your applicant commits to a school, they will be guided by the admissions office to fill out a lot of paperwork, often agree to a criminal background check that is mandated by the clinical settings where they will rotate in their third and fourth year, apply for institutional or federally guaranteed loans that have better terms than bank loans, and get the required health insurance, reports and vaccinations. Then there will be an orientation and your child, your medical student will be further along on the path to becoming a physician.

When they started college, you may have had to be told to leave after parent orientation, while you were handed a box of tissues. When medical school begins, the tables may turn. It will be time for you, the parent, guardian, friend, or mentor, to sit down with your medical student and say: *You know what honey? I got some news for you. Now you have to go. It's going to be difficult, you can handle it, and I'm going to be there with you every step of the way.*

On Children

As Kahlil Gibran cautioned parents in his beautiful poem:

On Children

Your children are not your children.

They are the sons and daughters of Life's longing for itself.

They come through you but not from you,

And though they are with you yet they belong not to you.

You may give them your love but not your thoughts,

For they have their own thoughts.

You may house their bodies but not their souls,

For their souls dwell in the house of tomorrow,

which you cannot visit, not even in your dreams...

~Kahlil Gibran

It's apt to remember that the premed soul dwells in the house of tomorrow, and even if you are a physician yourself, there is much of that dream that you can only hope to glimpse through your long relationship with your offspring.

What to Do If My Premed Doesn't Get In?

Luckily, because the application process is so long, it gives you a chance to prepare for disappointment. When an applicant does not get into medical school, they are in good company because over 50% of applicants are not accepted to medical school, and this should not be considered a reflection on them whatsoever.

When I worked at Cornell, I had access to an advisor database (AIS) generously provided by AAMC, that gave me detailed info about each Cornell student who had applied to medical school. One year, at the end of the application cycle, I decided to look at application outcomes for students who had near perfect grades and near perfect MCAT scores. There were six of these students; two of them had been accepted to many schools, two of them had no acceptances, and two of them received an acceptance from one medical school each. I found that very curious and it did confirm to me that schools are looking for things besides metrics. It's not a big surprise that the students who were not accepted to any medical school also had no clinical experience and few recent service activities on their applications. While they had a lot of research experience and they were very smart, they had not provided evidence that they knew what they were getting into when it came to medical school and joining a helping profession; they hadn't demonstrated that they cared about people and cared about the job of being a physician.

Often, applicants are discouraged by medical schools from applying in the following year because, medical schools reason, they need a year of doing something different and better to strengthen their applications. This can be frustrating. Surely they used those many months after applying to make themselves better applicants. By the time your student knows they are not getting into medical school (July), it's already getting late to apply in the current application cycle (we recommend that students submit their AMCAS application on the first day, in May). If your applicant has not received a single acceptance by the beginning of May and they are on some waitlists, they will need to decide whether to apply right then or wait through another cycle. A late application can doom their second cycle.

When an applicant is not accepted anywhere, they need to undertake an extensive comprehensive review of their application. They need to be willing to look at and hear about why they didn't get in and to strengthen the areas that are weak. Your premed can request feedback from their institutional advisor or even a kind soul at a medical school admissions office about how to strengthen their application, but the feedback is often general and hard to follow as clear guidance on how to proceed. It's really worth consulting with an independent advisor at that point, one who will give them the time to go over their application with a fine tooth comb.

Of course, go back through this book and evaluate whether your premed is strong in all the areas I covered. Your premed will need to take strategic action to strengthen key areas of their application and ensure that they better convey their medical school narrative the next time around.

Side Doors to a Medical Career

It's important to remember that there is more than one way to become a doctor and anyone who wants to become a doctor can, because there are many schools not in the continental United

States that are designed for people who they know will make good doctors but are not getting into America's allopathic or osteopathic schools. One such program is the University of Queensland Ochsner MD Program in Australia, a special program for American students with an outstanding residency match rate. Students study in Queensland for two years and then do clinical rotations in the U.S.

There are a handful of medical schools I recommend in the Caribbean, although it is really important to talk to someone knowledgeable about the quality of these programs. While many of these programs have acceptance rates up to 10 times higher than U.S. medical schools, programs in the Caribbean vary widely in quality, they are often for-profit institutions, and the residency match rate for international medical graduates is about 60 percent, compared with over 94 percent for U.S. graduates. It is harder to get residency as a graduate from a Caribbean school, but it's not impossible. American residency programs place a higher bar on graduates of foreign medical programs. Your student has to understand this and be absolutely committed to excelling in medical school to have a fair chance at residency placement.[19]

I also recommend the Atlantic Bridge Program that operates in Dublin, Ireland. There are other medical schools across Europe that accept American students but they don't necessarily have a program to match US students with US residencies or conduct classes in English; of course it would be fun to study in Italy, but remember that the instruction will be in Italian. While your premed may be accepted to a foreign medical school, if it doesn't have an official American medical instruction program (the ones I recommended above do), students are on their own when studying for American medical licensing exams.

---

19 https://www.nytimes.com/2021/06/29/health/caribbean-medical-school.html

Even this (not having an American program) isn't a dealbreaker. A young woman I worked with applied two years in a row to the Queensland Ochsner MD Program and didn't get in, so she decided to apply to their Australia-based medical program as a foreign student. She graduated from the program after four years and now she is working with an advisor to apply for a residency in the U.S.

Thoughts About Changing Direction

One of the beautiful things about raising and loving other human beings is our capacity for growth and change. People change. It's possible that at the end of the admissions cycle, your child has realized that they don't want to be a doctor and you, at age 45, have realized that you do! When these changes happen, you need to be in the present with them because these feelings may just be temporary and your premed may request a deferral. A deferral is usually not hard to get, but the applicant will need to have a good reason for their request, and cold feet is not a good reason. When your child does have that sense that this is not the right career for me, it's really important to be an open and honest listener, and trust their inner guidance.

About the Authors

Janet Snoyer is a medical school admissions advisor in private practice. She founded The Mentoring Alliance in 2013 after retiring from her position as Director of Prehealth Advising at Cornell University. During the coronavirus pandemic, she co-founded the HEAL Clinical Education Network, which provides problem-based seminars based on patient-consented, HIPAA-compliant video-recorded clinical encounters with real physicians and patients across several specialties. Janet is dedicated to promoting wellness among the premed population and in providing equitable access to expert advising for all applicants who seek it.

Elyse Perruchon studied biology and environmental studies at Oberlin College (2007). She brings her background in scientific inquiry and technical writing for an environmental consulting firm, and her experience as a patient care coordinator for a concierge integrative medical office, to help applicants reflect on and articulate the unique strengths, experiences, and goals they bring to the medical community. As an associate advisor and expert editor at The Mentoring Alliance, she works closely with Janet Snoyer to develop and implement a comprehensive application advising program and coach applicants throughout the application cycle.

www.premedadvisor.com
www.clinicalshadowing.com

www.ingramcontent.com/pod-product-compliance
Ingram Content Group UK Ltd.
Pitfield, Milton Keynes, MK11 3LW, UK
UKHW041634190726
13854UKWH00006B/2498